Alcoholic Liver Disease

Editors

NORMAN L. SUSSMAN
MICHAEL R. LUCEY

CLINICS IN LIVER DISEASE

www.liver.theclinics.com

Consulting Editor
NORMAN GITLIN

February 2019 • Volume 23 • Number 1

ELSEVIER

1600 John F. Kennedy Boulevard • Suite 1800 • Philadelphia, Pennsylvania, 19103-2899

http://www.theclinics.com

CLINICS IN LIVER DISEASE Volume 23, Number 1
February 2019 ISSN 1089-3261, ISBN-13: 978-0-323-65451-7

Editor: Kerry Holland
Developmental Editor: Meredith Madeira

Clinics in Liver Disease (ISSN 1089-3261) is published quarterly by Elsevier Inc., 360 Park Avenue South, New York, NY 10010-1710. Months of issue are February, May, August, and November. Business and Editorial Offices: 1600 John F. Kennedy Blvd., Ste. 1800, Philadelphia, PA 19103-2899. Customer Service Office: 3251 Riverport Lane, Maryland Heights, MO 63043. Periodicals postage paid at New York, NY and additional mailing offices. Subscription prices are $304.00 per year (U.S. individuals), $100.00 per year (U.S. student/resident), $542.00 per year (U.S. institutions), $409.00 per year (international individuals), $200.00 per year (international student/resident), $672.00 per year (international instituitions), $343.00 per year (Canadian individuals), $200.00 per year (Canadian student/resident), and $672.00 per year (Canadian institutions). Foreign air speed delivery is included in all *Clinics* subscription prices. All prices are subject to change without notice. **POSTMASTER:** Send address changes to *Clinics in Liver Disease*, Elsevier Health Sciences Division, Subscription Customer Service, 3251 Riverport Lane, Maryland Heights, MO 63043. **Customer Service: Telephone: 1-800-654-2452 (U.S. and Canada); 314-447-8871 (outside U.S. and Canada). Fax: 314-447-8029. E-mail: journalscustomer service-usa@elsevier.com (for print support); journalsonlinesupport-usa@elsevier.com (for online support).**

Reprints. For copies of 100 or more of articles in this publication, please contact the Commercial Reprints Department, Elsevier Inc., 360 Park Avenue South, New York, NY 10010-1710. Tel.: 212-633-3874; Fax: 212-633-3820; E-mail: reprints@elsevier.com.

Clinics in Liver Disease is covered in *MEDLINE/PubMed (Index Medicus)*, Science Citation Index Expanded, Journal Citation Reports/Science Edition, and Current Contents/Clinical Medicine.

Contributors

CONSULTING EDITOR

NORMAN GITLIN, MD, FRCP (LONDON), FRCPE (EDINBURGH), FAASLD, FACP, FACG
Head of Hepatology, Southern California Liver Centers, San Clemente, California, USA

EDITORS

NORMAN L. SUSSMAN, MD, FAASLD
Associate Professor, Medicine and Surgery, Baylor College of Medicine, Houston, Texas, USA

MICHAEL R. LUCEY, MD, FAASLD
Professor of Medicine and Surgery, Chief, Division of Gastroenterology and Hepatology, University of Wisconsin-Madison School of Medicine and Public Health, Madison, Wisconsin, USA

AUTHORS

PAGE D. AXLEY, MD
Resident in Internal Medicine, Department of Medicine, The University of Alabama at Birmingham, Birmingham, Alabama, USA

MAYA BALAKRISHNAN, MD, MPH
Assistant Professor, Section of Gastroenterology, Department of Medicine, Baylor College of Medicine, Houston, Texas, USA

ELIZABETH L. GODFREY, BSBE
MD Candidate, Department of Student Affairs, Baylor College of Medicine, Houston, Texas, USA

NADIA HAMMOUD, MD
Resident Physician, Department of Neurology, Baylor College of Medicine, Houston, Texas, USA

GENE Y. IM, MD
Assistant Professor of Medicine, Division of Liver Diseases, Icahn School of Medicine at Mount Sinai, Recanati-Miller Transplantation Institute, New York, New York, USA

JOOHI JIMENEZ-SHAHED, MD
Associate Professor of Neurology, Parkinson's Disease Center and Movement Disorders Clinic, Baylor College of Medicine, Houston, Texas, USA

FASIHA KANWAL, MD, MSHS
Professor, Section of Gastroenterology and Hepatology, Center for Innovations in Quality, Effectiveness and Safety (IQuESt), Michael E. DeBakey VA Medical Center, Section of Health Services Research, Department of Medicine, Baylor College of Medicine, Houston, Texas, USA

SAIRA AIJAZ KHADERI, MD, MPH
Assistant Professor of Surgery, Division of Abdominal Transplantation, Baylor College of Medicine, Houston, Texas, USA

THEMISTOKLIS KOURKOUMPETIS, MD
Department of Gastroenterology, Baylor College of Medicine, Houston, Texas, USA

MICHAEL R. LUCEY, MD, FAASLD
Professor of Medicine and Surgery, Chief, Division of Gastroenterology and Hepatology, University of Wisconsin-Madison School of Medicine and Public Health, Madison, Wisconsin, USA

JESSICA L. MELLINGER, MD, MSc
Clinical Lecturer, Division of Gastroenterology and Hepatology, Michigan Medicine, Ann Arbor, Michigan, USA

TAMIR MILOH, MD
Department of Pediatrics, Texas Children's Hospital, Houston, Texas, USA

TIMOTHY R. MORGAN, MD
Gastroenterology Section, VA Long Beach Healthcare System, Long Beach, California, USA

YAMINI NATARAJAN, MD
Assistant Professor, Section of Gastroenterology and Hepatology, Michael E. DeBakey VA Medical Center, Baylor College of Medicine, Houston, Texas, USA

STEPHEN CHRIS PAPPAS, MD, JD, FCLM, FAASLD
Associate Professor, Section of Gastroenterology, Department of Medicine, Baylor College of Medicine, Houston, Texas, USA

JIA QIN, MD, PhD
Department of Pathology, The Department of Veteran Affairs New York Harbor Healthcare System, Brooklyn, New York, USA

ABBAS RANA, MD
Assistant Professor, Division of Abdominal Transplantation, Department of Surgery, Baylor College of Medicine, Houston, Texas, USA

CRIT TAYLOR RICHARDSON, MD
Fellow in Gastroenterology, Division of Gastroenterology and Hepatology, University of Alabama at Birmingham, Birmingham, Alabama, USA

NITZAN C. ROTH, MD, PhD
Sandra Atlas Bass Center for Liver Diseases, Department of Medicine, Northwell Health, Manhasset, New York, USA

ASHWANI K. SINGAL, MD, MS, FACG, FAASLD
Associate Professor of Medicine, Director, Porphyria Center, Division of Gastroenterology and Hepatology, University of Alabama at Birmingham, Birmingham, Alabama, USA

GAGAN SOOD, MD, FAASLD
Department of Surgery, Division of Abdominal Transplantation, Baylor College of
Medicine, Houston, Texas, USA

RISE STRIBLING, MD
Associate Professor, Division of Abdominal Transplantation, Department of Surgery,
Baylor College of Medicine, Houston, Texas, USA

BRETT STYSKEL, MD
Medical Resident, Section of Gastroenterology and Hepatology, Michael E. DeBakey
VA Medical Center, Baylor College of Medicine, Houston, Texas, USA

VINAY SUNDARAM, MD, MSc
Department of Medicine, Comprehensive Transplant Center, Cedars-Sinai Medical
Center, Los Angeles, California, USA

SHARONDA ALSTON TAYLOR, MD
Department of Pediatrics, Texas Children's Hospital, Houston, Texas, USA

GERALD SCOTT WINDER, MD, MSc
Clinical Assistant Professor, Department of Psychiatry, Michigan Medicine, Ann Arbor,
Michigan, USA

Contents

in terms of disability-adjusted life years, an increase of more than 25% from 1990 to 2016. Understanding the epidemiology of alcoholic liver disease, including the regional variations in consumption and public policy, is an area of active research. In countries where the per capita consumption of alcohol decreases, there appears to be an associated decrease in disease burden. Given alcohol's health burden, an increased focus on alcohol control policies is needed.

Alcohol use is common during adolescence. Adolescent alcohol use is a global problem. The risk of alcohol dependence increases based on genetic and psychosocial factors. If a provider is concerned about use of alcohol, screening is recommended. From a public health perspective, alcohol abuse should be addressed.

Alcohol use disorder (AUD) is common in alcoholic liver disease (ALD) and intrinsic to its pathophysiology. Optimal treatment requires a multidisciplinary team approach and a working alliance between patients and providers. Diagnosing AUD involves a combination of thorough history taking, physical examination, screening questionnaires, and alcohol biomarkers. Alcohol biomarkers have advantages and limitations of use of which clinicians should be aware. AUD treatment is effective, multifaceted, and can be tailored to each individual. Available treatment modalities are myriad: motivational enhancement therapy, cognitive behavior therapy, 12-step facilitation, group therapies, intensive outpatient programs, inpatient and residential treatment, and relapse prevention medications.

Apart from the classic knowledge that ethanol mediates its hepatotoxicity through its metabolism to acetaldehyde, a well-known hepatotoxic molecule, recent research has elucidated several key mechanisms that potentiate ethanol's damage to the liver parenchyma, such as generation of free radicals, activation of Kupffer cells, and alterations to the human bacterial and fungal microbiome. Genetic studies have suggested the role of PNPLA3 and TM6SF2 gene mutations in the progression of alcoholic liver disease.

Alcoholic hepatitis is a unique type of alcohol-associated liver disease characterized by acute liver inflammation caused by prolonged heavy alcohol use. Treatment is mostly supportive. The short-term prognosis of acute alcoholic hepatitis depends on liver recovery, and ranges widely from rapid improvement to grim multiorgan failure despite treatment.

Refinement of scoring systems have enhanced prognostication to guide clinical decision making in alcoholic hepatitis. Recent advances in the treatment of alcoholic hepatitis have solidified corticosteroids as the cornerstone of treatment to enhance short-term survival, but not intermediate or long-term survival.

Malnutrition is a change in body composition owing to disordered nutrition associated with a decrease in function and poor clinical outcomes. Malnutrition can result from overnutrition, undernutrition and inflammatory activity. Patients with alcoholic liver disease are at increased risk for malnutrition. In this article, we discuss the different methods used to assess malnutrition, prevalence of malnutrition, potential mechanisms underlying malnutrition, and its treatments in patients with alcoholic liver disease.

Alcohol-associated cirrhosis (AC) contributes up to 50% of the overall cirrhosis burden in the United States. AC is typically a comorbid condition in association with alcohol-use disorder. AC is often coexistent with other conditions. Several noninvasive methods are available to assist in recognizing the presence of AC. The natural history of AC is governed by the patients continued drinking or abstinence. All treatment starts with abstinence. After decompensation, the progression to acute-on-chronic liver failure heralds death. When patients who have deteriorated are declined liver transplant, palliative care should be considered.

Alcoholic liver disease is a serious and increasing contributor to the global liver disease burden. Extensive selection criteria, including a minimum abstinence period, has previously been used to secure good outcomes but new research questions the effectiveness of abstinence periods and has recommended changes in integrated alcohol use treatment to effectively prevent relapse. Patients have unique health concerns, including posttransplantation risks of malignancy and metabolic complications, but overall very good long-term outcomes. Severe alcoholic hepatitis has been increasingly treated with early transplantation without a set sobriety period, with overall favorable outcomes, even with respect to recidivism.

Chronic alcohol use induces silent changes in the structure and function of the central and peripheral nervous systems that eventually result in irreversible, debilitating repercussions. Once identified, nutritional supplementation and cessation measures are critical in preventing further neurologic damage. The proposed mechanisms of neuronal injury in chronic alcohol abuse include direct toxic effects of alcohol and indirect effects, including those resulting from hepatic dysfunction, nutritional deficiencies, and neuroinflammation. Clinical manifestations include cerebellar ataxia, peripheral neuropathy and Wernicke-Korsakoff encephalopathy. Continued exploration of the pathophysiologic mechanisms may lead to the discovery of early interventions that can prevent permanent neurologic injury.

Hepatic steatosis and steatohepatitis have several etiologies; the most common are alcoholic steatohepatitis (ASH) and obesity/metabolic syndrome–induced steatohepatitis, also known as nonalcoholic steatohepatitis (NASH). Although the etiology of these 2 conditions is different, they share pathways to disease progression and severity. They also have differences in physiologic pathways, and shared and divergent mechanisms can be therapeutic targets. There is no approved pharmacologic therapy for NASH, but several molecules are under study. Focus remains on modulation of insulin resistance, oxidative stress, the inflammatory cascade, hepatic fibrosis, and cell death. This review provides an overview of pathophysiologic similarities and differences between ASH and NASH.

CLINICS IN LIVER DISEASE

Preface
Alcohol and Alcoholic Liver Disease

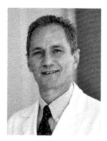
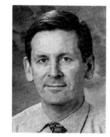

Norman L. Sussman, MD, FAASLD   Michael R. Lucey, MD, FAASLD
Editors

It's a great advantage not to drink among hard drinking people.
— F. Scott Fitzgerald, The Great Gatsby

Welcome to this issue of *Clinics in Liver Disease*, an issue devoted to alcohol. Alcohol was the first agent recognized as a cause of liver disease, and it remains synonymous with cirrhosis to the lay public. Alcohol has been touted as a panacea and reviled as a social and medical menace. It has been an important factor in medicine since Hippocratic times; a Medline search for "alcohol and liver disease" identified almost 37,000 citations from 1946 to 2018. The ill effects of alcohol extend beyond the liver, but we have taken a fairly liver-focused view: this is *Clinics in LIVER Disease*, after all.

We enjoyed the opportunity to assemble a talented and enthusiastic group of authors who contributed a total of 13 articles. Our hope was to highlight important issues and stimulate discussion on the place of alcohol in contemporary medicine. We start with an unusual nonmedical topic, a history of alcohol in ancient and modern civilizations. We then move on to a wide range of issues that confront practitioners who deal with alcohol-related problems. The subsequent articles include pathology, legal issues, epidemiology and population health, pediatric issues, alcohol use disorder, genetics, acute alcoholic hepatitis, nutrition, cirrhosis, alcohol-related diseases of the central nervous system, and potential future therapies that may emerge from studies in nonalcoholic fatty liver disease. We hope that students and professionals who study alcoholic liver disease will find useful opinions and challenging ideas in the pages of this issue.

We would like to thank the authors who did the difficult work and submitted outstanding articles on time. We also wish to thank the editorial staff at Elsevier,

Clin Liver Dis 23 (2019) xiii–xiv
https://doi.org/10.1016/j.cld.2018.10.001
1089-3261/19/© 2018 Published by Elsevier Inc.

liver.theclinics.com

who kept us on track to get this issue out on time. Finally, we would like to thank Norman Gitlin, MD, who gave us the opportunity to edit this issue of *Clinics in Liver Disease*.

Norman L. Sussman, MD, FAASLD
Medicine and Surgery
Baylor College of Medicine
6620 Main Street, Suite 1425
Houston, TX 77030, USA

Michael R. Lucey, MD, FAASLD
Medicine and Surgery
University of Wisconsin-Madison School of Medicine and Public Health
600 Highland Avenue
Madison, WI 53792, USA

E-mail addresses:
normans@bcm.edu (N.L. Sussman)
mrl@medicine.wisc.edu (M.R. Lucey)

Introduction
Alcohol and Alcoholism

Saira Aijaz Khaderi, MD, MPH

KEYWORDS

- Alcohol • Alcoholism • History of alcoholic beverages

KEY POINTS

- The first evidence of alcoholic drinks dates back to the prehistory era, after humans established sedentary communities.
- Winemaking and breweries were a stimulus to civilization in early history.
- Wine played an important role in the rituals of Judaism and Christianity, but was forbidden in Islam.
- The pilgrims brought imported wines and the skill of brewing alcohol to the New World.

"The bulk of this chapter is an abbreviated version of the excellent book by Ian Gately, "Drink: A Cultural History of Alcohol". Those interested are encouraged to read the book in its entirety."

PREHISTORY

The first definite evidence of the preparation of alcoholic drinks appeared around 8000 BC after humans took up agriculture and established sedentary communities. The earliest proof comes from chemical analysis of residues inside pottery jars found in Jiahu, North China. Dating back to 7000 to 6600 BC, these clay vessels contained a fermented drink made with rice, honey, grapes, and hawthorn berries.

Evidence that plants were being cultivated to manufacture alcohol first appeared in the Fertile Crescent, a geographic area curving between the Mediterranean and the Persian Gulf. Analysis of a yellow residue found in a jar at a Neolithic settlement in Haji Firuz Tepe (present-day Iran) dating back to 5400 to 5000 BC revealed the jar had once held wine. Several houses in the same village had multiple similar vessels suggesting it was a significant staple of their diet. Winemaking was the best method for storing highly perishable grapes in such communities, but whether the resultant fluid was meant for nutrition or intoxication remains unknown. These same inhabitants

The author has nothing to disclose.
Division of Abdominal Transplantation, Baylor College of Medicine, 6620 Main Street, Suite 1450, Houston, TX 77030, USA
E-mail address: Saira.Khaderi@bcm.edu

Clin Liver Dis 23 (2019) 1–10
https://doi.org/10.1016/j.cld.2018.09.009
1089-3261/19/© 2018 Elsevier Inc. All rights reserved.

were also likely making mead from honey and beer from surplus grain. The first proof that beer was being brewed in this area comes from residue found in a pottery vessel in the Zagros Mountains of Iran dating to 3100 to 2900 BC.

By the middle of the third millennium it was clear that alcohol was more than sustenance to the people of the Fertile Crescent. In Sumer, located at the confluence of the rivers Tigris and Euphrates, art and writing were used to record the social roles played by alcohol. In Uruk, the largest city in Sumer (and possibly the world) at that time, beer was produced on an epic scale. The Sumerians documented the number and types of beer they brewed: eight from barley, eight from wheat, and three from mixed types of grains. Laws incised on clay tablets taught us they had regulated drinking places and artifacts suggested that beer was a favorite of the elite and was offered to the Gods. Characters in the epic Sumerian poem Gilgamesh (c. 2000 BC) drank water during their usual daily tasks but resorted to alcohol when they were celebrating. Intoxication was common in their new year festivities. The highlight was a ceremonial and public act of coitus between the king and Ishtar, the goddess of procreation. The mythical coupling was believed to have resulted in Ninkasi, the goddess of brewing.

EGYPT

The Egyptian story of drinking begins in the city of Hierakonpolis where ruins contain evidence of the world's oldest brewery dating back to 3400 BC. The brewery was capable of producing up to 300 gallons of beer per day. Hierakonpolis was also the site of a thriving pottery industry whose primary products were jugs and cups used for drinking beer. The abundance of such items, and the relative scale of the brewing operations, suggested that beer was a vital part of this community. Commoners drank beer and rulers preferred wine, an imported luxury and symbol of power. King Scorpion's tomb held approximately 700 wine jars, most of which did not originate in Egypt. The presence of so many imported jars suggested the art of winemaking had spread throughout the region and that wine trade was a stimulus to civilization in the area.

By 3100 BC, beer was established as a beverage for the working class and wine was the drink of the elite. Papyrus scrolls bearing financial accounts reported the laborers who built the pyramids of the Giza plateau were provided a daily ration of one and a third gallons of beer. At 5% alcohol by volume, the pyramids were essentially built by an army of drunks.

GREECE

Wine production reached the Hellenic peninsula by 2000 BC and was commonplace in Classical Greece by 1700 BC. The Greeks were the first civilization to leave a coherent account of their thoughts on alcohol, both its advantages and detriments. Wine was ubiquitous in Hellenic civilization. It was used as an offering to the Gods, as a currency to buy imports from distant countries, as a part of rituals, as a medicine, and to quench thirst.

In Athens, consumption of wine was considered a civic duty. Officials oversaw its distribution at annual feasts and ensured that all present received their fair share. Such equality of portions eventually planted the seed for *demokratia* or "people power." Athens was also the principal source of inspiration during Greece's classical age. Acknowledged by its peers as the leader in cultural matters, poets, playwrights, politicians, and philosophers in Athens set down their feelings about wine. Wine was considered a force for good, a substance that enabled people to relax while elevating their minds.

The Greeks were discriminatory drinkers and believed that certain vineyards had been blessed with magical soil. Some vineyards produced wine with sensational flavors, whereas wine from other vineyards produced undesirable side effects. For example, the wine of Heraea in Arcadia was known to "drive men out of their senses and make women inclined to pregnancy." There were also special wines for loosening the bowels, sweetening breath, and for healing wounds and cancers.

The tendency of drinking to cause a hangover was noted in Greek literature. The poet Philyllius believed the key to avoiding a hangover was drinking good quality wine. Boiled cabbage was the best way to clear a fuzzy head associated with a hangover, but some drinkers believed the cure was more painful than the ailment. The usual way to recover was to sleep it off but sleeping late eventually came to be known as the hallmark of the drunkard.

The Greeks believed drinking to be an inherently pleasurable activity. It was understandable that people would want to indulge in it as much as possible. Those who indulged too frequently were considered weak, succumbing to an entirely natural impulse. However, sobriety was thought to be highly suspicious. Sober people were believed to be coldhearted and earned the title "water drinkers." Water drinkers were believed to lack passion and exuded a noxious odor.

The Greeks recognized the potentially dangerous effects of alcohol. Severe intoxication was believed to be a possession during which a spirit took command of the drinker's reasoning and forced them to reveal their secrets. The Greeks attributed the hazardous effects of alcohol with the Greek god Dionysus. According to legend, Dionysus had been offered a drink of goat's milk from a man named Ikarios during one of his travels. To return the favor, Dionysus presented Ikarios with vines and directions on how to cultivate them and turn the fruit into wine creating the first Greek vintage. Soon neighbors were dancing in the streets praising the new drink until one by one, they lost control of their legs. Ikarios was accused of poisoning the people and beaten to death, his mutilated body thrown into a well. His daughter went mad, hung herself, and was turned into a star in the constellation of Virgo. Her dog, Maira, never forgave humanity for the death of her mistress and she is said to rule over the hottest days of summer. Like wine, Dionysus brought happiness but also chaos and misery.

Greeks had strict rules about who could drink wine. It was not customary for women to drink. With a few rare exceptions, women were expected to steer clear of drinking because wine made them *paroinos* (violent when drunk). With regards to age, Plato proposed a minimum drinking age of 18 in his *Laws*, a framework for the legislation of an ideal society. According to Plato, the young had "excitable" dispositions and allowing them to drink would "pour fire upon fire." In *Republic*, a revised blueprint for the ideal state, Plato changed his mind about the minimum drinking age. Because wine was a necessary part of culture, he believed it was best that young men gained early experience of its effects so they could learn how to manage it. The *symposium* was a formal drinking party attended only by men and the perfect forum for training youth on how to manage their alcohol. Unfortunately, after an evening of dinner, sensible drinking, and entertainment, many of the symposia ended in riot and disorder.

ROME

The Romans were the next great drinking civilization to emerge in the classical world. Rome was almost completely dry in the early years. When the followers of Dionysus reached the Roman territory in the second century BC, they were met with suspicion. People congregating in large groups for the purpose of becoming drunk did not make sense to this sober society. The Romans decided it was all a part of a sinister plot to overthrow their rule. Soon afterward, all the Dionysus shrines were destroyed and nearly 7000 Dionysus followers were slaughtered.

It was only a few decades later that the Roman attitude toward drinking vastly changed. Wine was part of the rations of Roman legionaries and an increasing supply was necessary to support the efforts of growing armies. In 160 BC, the Roman senate ordered the translation of *De Agri Cultura*, a Carthaginian book on viticulture. With every aspect of vineyard management addressed in the book, *De Agri Cultura* was circulated among landowners and Rome quickly became a significant producer of wine. The new vineyards were large commercial ventures that focused on producing bulk wine. The increase in supply helped alter the Romans thoughts on alcohol. It led to Romans adopting the drinking culture of the Greeks. By the middle of the first century BC, Rome had transformed from a sober society to a major producer with both discriminatory and populated drinkers.

As the Roman Empire spread throughout the Mediterranean region, traditional Roman values were replaced by heavy drinking, ambition, and corruption. The decadent style of drinking was nowhere more evident than in Pompeii, the center of the Roman wine trade. Pompeiians would cook themselves in the municipal baths to sweat out previous binges, then, "without putting on a stitch of clothing, still naked and gasping, [would] seize hold of a huge jar…and, as if to demonstrate their strength, pour down the entire contents…vomit it up again immediately, and then drink another jar." By the second and first centuries BC, intoxication was common and prominent men of affairs were praised for their moderation in drinking. This was likely a backlash to the growing misuse of alcohol in society.

JUDAISM

The connection of the Jews to viticulture was reflected in their sacred texts. Wine made its debut in the Tanakh with Noah. After the flood, Noah disembarked from his ark and planted a vineyard, and "he drank of the wine, and was drunken, and was uncovered in his tent." The prophets of the Tanakh discussed the consumption of wine and the Book of Isaiah provided practical advice as to the best way to lay out a vineyard.

Wine also played an important role in the personal rituals of the Jews. The weekly Sabbath included a prayer delivered over a cup of wine, and circumcisions, weddings, and funerals were all celebrated with the consumption of wine.

CHRISTIANITY

Christianity arose in the first century AD in Roman Judea. The rapid dissemination of Christianity was a consequence of the responsibility Christ laid on his followers to spread the message. In Christianity, not only could wine relieve thirst and inspire joy, but it might also represent the substantiated blood of the son of God. Christ made this potential apparent to his disciples at the last supper. After filling his cup with wine and sharing it, he explained the significance of the act, "And he took the cup, and when he had given thanks, he gave it to them and they all drank of it. And he said unto them, This is my blood of the new testament which is shed for man." (Mark 14:23–25) So pervasive was wine in the teachings of the new religion, the apostle Paul believed it necessary to make clear that wine's role was principally symbolic; the Eucharist, a ceremony where patrons gathered to share bread and wine, was not an invitation to gluttony or drunkenness. Paul considered wine to be a creation of God and inherently good. Its use for medicinal purposes was recommended but intoxication was condemned. Those who could not control their drinking were recommended to completely abstain.

ISLAM

Islam, the revelation of Allah via his prophet Muhammad, was born in the middle of the first millennium AD. The basic concepts of the new religion were simple: to acknowledge only one God (Allah), pray five times a day, fast each year, to give alms, and make a pilgrimage to Mecca once in a lifetime. Further instructions on how to live as a Muslim were provided in the Quran, the word of God spoken to his prophet. Born in a region of drinkers, Islam's attitude toward drinking changed from approval into condemnation over time. Alcohol was initially mentioned in the Quran as a good thing alongside water, milk, and honey. By its next appearance its status was equivocal, "In them is great sin and some profit, for men; but the sin is greater than the profit." Despite the news that drinking was sinful, many faithful continued to drink and some would not sober up for prayers. The prophet consulted his god and was advised that no Muslim could attend prayers if drunk. Given five prayers throughout the day, this could be interpreted as a de facto ban. However, Arabs continued to drink and it was not until a bloody affair that a third consultation led to complete prohibition, "Strong drink, games of chance, idols and divining arrows are an abomination of Satan; avoid them, that you might prosper," for "Satan's plan is to excite enmity and hatred between you, with intoxicants and gambling, and hinder you from the remembrance of Allah and from prayer: Will ye not then abstain?"

Islam set about to conquer the drinking world and within 100 years of the prophet's death, Muslims controlled Egypt, North Africa, most of the Persian Empire, Sicily, Corsica, Spain, Portugal, and parts of France. New subjects who converted immediately gained the privileges and duties of being Muslim. Non-Muslims paid a poll tax, were allowed to continue drinking, and to produce and sell wine to each other for sacred and secular purposes. Taverns continued to operate but were forbidden to serve Muslims.

While Christian Europe was in the Dark Ages, Muslim scientists picked up where the Greeks had left off and made substantial contributions to medicine, physics, mathematics, astronomy, and chemistry. Although it was Aristotle who had worked out the process of distillation, it was the Muslims who perfected its practice and who managed to extract alcohol from wine. Jabir Ibn Hayyan (721–815), the father of the science of chemistry, established the science of identifying substances by their properties and invented techniques and equipment for isolating them.

Muslims also contributed to mankind's understanding of the effects of alcohol on the human body. Al Zahrawi was Islam's greatest surgeon. Despite working in a society where alcohol was prohibited, he had sufficient patients to identify its detrimental effects. Al Zahrawi said alcohol could cause convulsions, apoplexy, dementia, partial and total paralysis, difficulties in articulation, gout, and "disturbances of the liver."

Islam lost a potentially useful ally when Prince Vladimir of Kiev, whose kingdom formed modern day Russia, chose Christianity for his subjects. A religion that required circumcision, ate no pork, and drank no wine was not agreeable to Vladimir's lifestyle. The Dark Ages in Europe ended, and Europeans started to push Islam out of their continent.

CHRISTIAN EUROPE

The Crusades were a series of religious and political wars fought between the Christians and Muslims for control of the Holy Land. Pope Urban II called on all good Christians to aid the Christian Byzantine Empire, which was under attack by the Muslim Turks. Anyone who answered the call was given complete remission of his sins.

When the crusaders returned home, they were surrounded by limitless opportunities to indulge in alcohol. Everyone in Europe drank and drank several times a day. The amount and type of alcohol one consumed was dependent on their caste: clergy, nobility, or commoners.

The clergy drank the least, but they were all required to drink wine daily in memory of their Savior. To ensure ample supply, the clergy cultivated the grape wherever climate permitted. The monks of the Cistercians led the field of viticulture and were rewarded for their prayers with the best vineyards in the region, which they turned into laboratories. They studied in detail the vintages that each produced and paid special attention to the soil. Once a monastery had 60 monks, 12 of them were required to leave and to found a new one. There were 400 Cistercian monasteries by 1153 AD and 2000 a century later.

The nobles consumed the most amount of wine, great even in comparison with the wine lovers of Pompeii. Excess was the hallmark for those at the pinnacle of feudal society. Magnificent clothes, ostentatious palaces, exotic entertainment, and excessive alcohol intake was the hallmark of high society. Imported wine, which was expensive and therefore noble, started a viticultural revolution in the Bordeaux region of France. By the first quarter of the thirteenth century, Bordeaux was exporting about 20,000 tons of wine per year to England. In the true spirit of excess, King Edward II ordered the equivalent of 1,152,000 bottles of wine for his wedding celebration. The population of London, where the wedding took place, was less than 80,000 at the time.

Commoners, the third category of the English feudal system, drank ale. Adults and children drank ale several times a day, with breakfast, lunch, and before bedtime. A gallon per head per day was the standard ration. Ale was the only safe, commonly available drink and a large amount provided them with sufficient calories. Given the crowded and unsanitary conditions, water had a bad reputation of being a carrier of disease and was frequently avoided.

DISTILLATION

Arnald of Villanova (d. 1315) was a physician and alchemist who promoted the use of alcohol as a cure for any ailment. He believed that wine was suited for every age and blessed everyone with good health. He experimented with the science of distillation and named distilled spirits *aqua vitae* (water of life). Distillation first flourished in Germany and, by the fifteenth century, apothecaries would sell spirits by shots to the public as a health tonic. They were retailed as *brandy*, which was derived from the German translation for "burned wine." Hieronymus Braunschweig, a German physician, wrote the *Big Book of Distillation* praising the medicinal benefits of distilled spirits. He wrote, "It eases diseases coming of cold. It comforts the heart. It heals all old and new sores on the head. It causes good color in a person…it eases the pain in the teeth and causes sweet breath…it heals the short-winded. It causes good digestion and appetite…and takes away belching. It eases the yellow jaundice, the dropsy, the gout, the pain in breasts when they be swollen, and heals all diseases in the bladder…It heals the bites of a mad dog."

THE AMERICAS

In 1492, the Spanish king and queen, Ferdinand and Isabella, financed a fleet of ships that sailed across the Atlantic to the Americas. Within 50 years, the Spanish conquered the Incan and Aztec civilizations and established an empire that stretched from Florida to southern Chile. The Mesoamerican civilizations, between Mexico and Panama, were the most ingenious in identifying potential sources of alcohol.

The manufacturing of alcoholic beverages from cacti was widespread among hunter-gatherer tribes. Tribes would move to areas where cacti were in fruit, spend their time brewing and drinking, and then move on to the next location when the season was complete. One such tribe, the Chichimeca of central Mexico were noted by the Spanish to be highly volatile when drunk. The women would hide the menfolk's bows and arrows to prevent any untimely deaths. Interestingly, the Chichimeca never all got drunk at the same time. They appointed drink monitors whose duty it was to keep a good lookout and stay sober.

Maize, the principal cereal crop of the Americas, was fermented to make *tesguino* (maize beer) and *balche*, mead fermented with the bark of the balche tree. Although many of the native types of alcoholic drinks fell out of use after the Spanish conquest, *pulque*, the fermented sap of *maguey* (the agave plant), grew in popularity. The manufacturing of pulque was complex and required the death of the plant. Magueys mature when the center begins to swell and sends out a single flower stalk. The flower bud is cut and the cavity is scraped clean, which then fills with sap. The sap is extracted two to three times a day, and a large plant can yield up to 7 L per day. The plant can live in this wounded state for 6 months producing up to 1000 L.

The Spanish tried their best to exterminate Aztec and other New World religious practices and to replace them with Christianity. This cultural transformation resulted in an increase in drunkenness among their new subjects. It is likely that most of them resorted to alcohol when they were forced into unpleasant living conditions. Although the indigenous people continued with their traditional brews postconquest, the Spanish introduced their distilled spirits and wine.

PILGRIMS

The decision to establish English colonies in the Americas was heavily influenced by the success of the Spanish in the New World domains. In 1584, Sir Walter Raleigh received letters patent from Queen Elizabeth for the foundation of an American colony. The first scouts returned within a few months and described the new land with an abundance of vines. Every tree seemed to be draped with vines and the native tribes were friendly, sober, and preferred water. Unlike their neighbors in Central and South America, the North American natives did not drink alcohol.

A group of English Protestants taking refuge in the Dutch town of Leyden decided to attempt a colony in North America where they may practice their religion freely. They had read of the damage water drinking had reeked on previous voyages and included a vast store of alcohol in their provisions. Under the leadership of John Carver, more than 100 pilgrims and 36 sailors set out on a transatlantic voyage on the Mayflower. They landed near Cape Cod in November 1620. The landscape was wild and forbidding and their sense of isolation grew when they started to explore their new home.

Winter was approaching, and the pilgrims settled where they were because resources were running scarce, especially their beer. Epidemics broke out among the pilgrims and mariners, but the stock of beer was not offered to the sick for fear the supply would not be enough for the journey home. William Bradford, chosen to lead the colonists after the death of John Carver, reported: "As this calamity fell…the passengers that were to be left here to plant…were hasted ashore and made to drink water that the seamen might have the more beer, and one [Bradford himself] in his sickness desiring but a small can of beer, it was answered that if he was their own father he should have none."

When spring arrived, there were only 53 pilgrims still alive. The *Mayflower* returned to England in 1621 and the colonists continued to explore the new land. They met an

English-speaking Indian named Samoset who had picked up the language from passing fisherman and slave traders. Samoset introduced the pilgrims to neighboring tribes and peace and harmony were agreed among them. Over the next two decades, the colonists flourished and became self-sufficient in food and trade. In addition to imported liquor, surplus food was used to make home brews resulting in plenty of booze in the colonies. By 1634 every community in New England was required by law to build an ordinarie, an inn built for "the receiving, refreshment, and entertainment of travelers and strangers, and to serve public occasions." Ordinaries sold local brews, imported wines and spirits, and their prices were fixed by law.

The pilgrims had planned their colony while in Holland and had sent for their families and friends once the colonies were established and prospering. The Dutch had a good picture of the progress of the English and realized that Europeans could prosper in the Americas. They formed the West India Company (1621), which established colonies near the Delaware River and in 1625 purchased Manhattan Island from the its native American owners.

Henry Hudson, who was exploring the region in 1609, had met some Indians on the island in the river that bears his name. As was custom of that time, he offered them a drink, but the Indians did not like its smell and refused. One of their warriors, not wanting to appear ill mannered, accepted the offer and collapsed on the spot after swallowing the entire drink in one gulp. He rose up soon afterward and declared the drink to be wonderful. The rest of the group followed the lead of their friend and drank to the point of intoxication. Once the indigenous people had their first taste of alcohol, they seemed eager to make up for lost time. They seemed incapable of drinking for any other reason but to get drunk as quickly as possible. Drunkenness often led to violence and, after observing the effects of alcohol on the native people, the colonists were no longer so free with their liquor. The problem was exacerbated by the abundance of spirits in the Americas. Their concentrated form made them easier to carry across the Atlantic and, unlike most Europeans who started drinking beer or wine when they were children, frequently a native American's first drink was heavily concentrated liquor. They looked to alcohol more for stimulation rather than refreshment and many quickly ruined themselves on the white man's "wicked water."

CHAMPAGNE

The wine from the Champagne district of France was a still, sweet drink with a gold-tinted red. It was all the rage at the French court when King Charles II had lived there in exile. This fashionable French elixir was touted in England where it, too, became all the rage. The champagne the English came to know and love was different than the wine from the French court. It arrived in England every fall and was placed in cellars to sleep through winter. When the temperatures rose in spring, it underwent a secondary fermentation making it fizzy and dry. Although the French considered the bubbles to be sacrilege, in England they were fashionable. However, by the time champagne was sparkling in London, parts of English society turned against everything French. In 1679, imports of French wine were banned altogether.

RUM

Europeans had an insatiable appetite for sugar. Sugar for the English market was mostly produced in the Caribbean islands, which the English had colonized around the same time as New England. Molasses, a by-product of refined sugar, fermented readily and was an ideal raw material for distillation, and rum was born. By 1651 Barbados was the main source of molasses and, soon after rum made its debut, the crop covered much of the island. African slaves were brought over by the tens then hundreds of thousands to work on plantations in the New World. New Englanders started slaving in earnest once they realized that Caribbean rum commanded a premium in Africa. Over the next quarter century "about one in seven English slave voyages began in the Americas rather than in England." According to one estimate, they carried 1.3 million gallons of spirits to Africa between 1680 and 1713, which they exchanged for approximately 60,000 humans.

Africa was a seller's market and business was held on African terms or not at all. The principal demand was for cloth, but rum was second in line. Sub-Saharan Africa was populated by people who consumed alcohol for cultural and hedonistic purposes. Most religions in the area believed life to be a voyage by a soul from and back to the spirit world. Alcohol was used to ease each soul through conception, birth, puberty, and death. It was sprinkled over the forehead of newborns and on the earth covering a fresh grave. European merchants could not even do business with the Africans without first giving presents of rum.

GIN

In 1700 London was the largest metropolitan city in Europe. Affluence and poverty existed side by side and the wealthy were neighbors with the laborers. London was also one of the most exciting cities in Europe packed with places to drink including traditional inns, alehouses, and taverns. Beer was the people's choice and the average Englishman went through 75 gallons of beer every year. The British prided themselves on their drinking and foreigners marveled at their consumption, "Would you believe it, though water is to be had in abundance in London, and of fairly good quality, absolutely none is drunk? The lower classes, even the paupers, do not know what it is to quench their thirst with water. In this country nothing but beer is drunk…It is said that more grain is consumed in England for making beer than for making bread." The British drank hard but could hold their liquor and believed drunkenness was a benign condition. The 1720s, however, brought on a new kind of reckless drinking centered on the consumption of gin.

Gin was the English name for the Dutch *Genever*, a distilled spirit flavored with juniper. England had an excess of grain at that time and measures were necessary to increase the income of landowners. The "Act for the Encouraging of the Distillation of Brandy and Spirits from Corn" was passed, which allowed anyone in England to distil alcohol using English cereals. The act was hugely successful, and stills sprang up all over England. The new appetite for gin supported the general price of corn and used the damaged grain that bakers and brewers would not buy. Gin was sold everywhere, from prisons to crypts of churches to stalls at public executions. Gin was cheap and a quick way to get drunk.

In 1700, the average English adult drank a third of a gallon of gin per year. By 1723, every man, woman, and child in London drank more than a pint of gin per head per week. This high level of consumption led to extreme levels of drunkenness in the capitol. The gin craze, as it came to be known, was linked to a rising crime rate. The town was plagued by thieves and overrun with highwaymen. Condemned men would stop by at gin shops for a quick drink en route to the gallows. Even the hangmen were drunk sometimes. On one notorious occasion, a drunken executioner tried to hang the priest who was on the scaffold to deliver the last rites instead of the condemned.

THE DOWNFALL OF ALCOHOL

Consumption of alcohol peaked in the 1870s and then began a downward trend. Some historians believe the decline was related to the increasing caloric content provided by other foods, such as butter, sugar, and bacon. As the world became more industrialized, drunkenness was not consistent with a reliable workforce. During the second half of the eighteenth century many Protestant churches began to reject traditional Christian beliefs on alcohol and instead taught that alcohol was evil and drinking it was a sin. Over time more personal, economic, criminal, and family problems were attributed to alcohol. Temperance groups started by promoting voluntary temperance of the moderate use of alcohol but would soon demand mandatory and legally enforced prohibition. They insisted total prohibition would end poverty, violence, crime, marital conflict, and all other personal and societal problems. Instead prohibition in the United States led to largely negative economic effects. The closing of breweries, distilleries, and saloons led to the elimination of thousands of jobs and the federal government lost a total of $11 billion in lost tax revenue.

In 1935 Alcoholics Anonymous was created to address the problem of alcoholism, and in 1980 Mothers Against Drunk Driving was organized to reduce drunk driving and raise consciousness about the unacceptability of this crime. The last three decades have seen increasing calls for further restrictions on the availability and the consumption of alcohol.

Alcoholic drinks have been produced and consumed for thousands of years and played a pivotal role in religion, nutrition, and enhancing the quality and pleasures of life. Alcohol's place in society is controversial and will likely remain the subject of great debate for many years to come.

FURTHER READINGS

Gately I. Drink: A Cultural History of Alcohol. New York: Gotham Books; 2008.
Rogers A. Proof. New York: Mariner Books; 2014.

Histopathology of Alcohol-Related Liver Diseases

Nitzan C. Roth, MD, PhD[a],*, Jia Qin, MD, PhD[b,1]

KEYWORDS

- Alcohol-related liver disease • Alcoholic hepatitis • Alcoholic steatohepatitis
- Alcoholic foamy degeneration • Alcoholic fatty liver with cholestasis • Liver biopsy
- Histology

KEY POINTS

- Excessive alcohol consumption can lead to a spectrum of liver histopathology, including steatosis, steatohepatitis, foamy degeneration, fatty liver with cholestasis, and cirrhosis.
- The histologic severity of steatohepatitis does not correlate with its clinical severity, which can range from a total lack of symptoms to the clinical syndrome of alcohol-related hepatitis with rapid onset of jaundice and liver failure.
- Liver biopsy is not routinely recommended to ascertain a diagnosis of alcohol-related liver disease in patients with an uncertain alcohol history, because the histologic features of alcohol-related liver diseases can be found in other diseases, including nonalcoholic steatohepatitis or drug-induced liver injury.
- Although variability in sampling and pathologist interpretation are of some concern, liver biopsy remains the gold standard for distinguishing between steatohepatitis and noninflammatory histologic patterns of injury that can also cause the clinical syndrome of alcohol-related hepatitis.

INTRODUCTION

Histologic assessment of the liver by biopsy has, historically, been a cornerstone of the diagnosis and management of liver diseases. It is no coincidence that many of the giants of hepatology were themselves expert pathologists. For the modern clinician, liver biopsy "has three major roles: (1) for diagnosis, (2) for assessment of prognosis (disease staging), and/or (3) to assist in making therapeutic management

Disclosure Statement: The authors have nothing to disclose.
[a] Sandra Atlas Bass Center for Liver Diseases Department of Medicine Northwell Health, 400 Community Drive, Manhasset, NY 11030, USA; [b] Department of Pathology, The Department of Veteran Affairs New York Harbor Healthcare System, 800 Poly Place, Brooklyn, NY 11209, USA
[1] Present address: 188 East 93rd Street, Apartment 3K, New York, NY 10128.
* Corresponding author.
E-mail address: NRoth2@northwell.edu

decisions."[1] The role of liver biopsy in the diagnosis and management of alcohol-related liver diseases (ALDs) is controversial because of several factors, including limited available pharmacologic treatments of ALD; concerns about the costs, availability, and safety of biopsy; and the growing availability of noninvasive tools to assess steatosis and liver fibrosis. These factors have led to increased reliance on clinical diagnosis alone for many patients with ALD. The aims of this review are to describe the key histologic features of acute and chronic ALD and to provide some pearls and pitfalls for using liver biopsy in the diagnosis and management of ALD.

HISTOPATHOLOGY OF CHRONIC ALCOHOL-RELATED LIVER DISEASES

ALD encompasses a spectrum of injury, ranging from simple steatosis to severe inflammatory hepatitis and variable fibrosis from mild to cirrhosis. Early histologic evidence of liver injury in the form of steatosis is present in more than 90% of patients after even a few days of heavy drinking. Steatosis is defined by the presence of lipid droplets in the hepatocyte cytoplasm and is seen in a variety of liver diseases. In ALD, the steatosis begins in the centrilobular zone and progresses toward the periportal zone. It may begin with small lipid droplets (microvesicular steatosis) that can later enlarge and coalesce into large fat droplets that displace the nucleus to the periphery of the hepatocyte (macrovesicular steatosis [**Fig. 1**]). Large fat droplets can coalesce to form fat cysts, and continuing accumulation of fat may lead to rupture of a fat cyst with a histiocytic reaction, forming a lipogranuloma (see **Fig. 1**). Steatosis is graded by the percentage of hepatocytes containing lipid droplets, with less than or equal to 5% considered normal and greater than 5% considered pathologic (fatty degeneration). When more than half of hepatocytes have steatosis, fatty liver has developed. In simple steatosis, the centrilobular zone and portal tracts have no fibrosis or inflammatory infiltrates. Simple steatosis and fatty liver are reversible and rarely symptomatic.

In patients with alcohol-related fatty liver, years of continued heavy alcohol use (typically, >20 g or 1–2 standard drinks daily for women and >60 g or 3–4 standard drinks daily for men) can lead to progressive liver fibrosis and, eventually, cirrhosis; portal hypertension with its attendant complications; and an increased risk of liver cancer. Fibrosis in ALD begins in the centrilobular zone, with activation of stellate cells leading to collagen deposition surrounding the central venules and then extending into

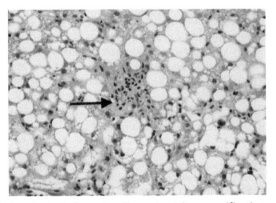

Fig. 1. Macrovesicular steatosis (hematoxylin-eosin stain, magnification ×40). The hepatocytes contain single large fat droplets that displace the hepatocyte's nucleus to its periphery. Prior rupture of a fat cyst has led to formation of a lipogranuloma (*arrow*) consisting of histiocytes and inflammatory cells surrounding small extracellular lipid droplets.

the perivenular sinusoids in a pericellular fashion, forming an arachnoid or chicken-wire pattern of fine collagen reticulum around individual hepatocytes (**Fig. 2**A). This pattern is best appreciated with use of a Masson trichrome stain or Sirius red stain that stains collagen bright blue or red, respectively. The fibrosis progresses and extends to the portal tracts followed by development of nonbridging fibrous septa or bridging fibrosis between adjacent central veins, from centrilobular to periportal zones, and between adjacent portal tracts (see **Fig. 2**B). Finally, if the alcohol-related injury continues, complete fibrous septa form and enclose regenerative nodules, defining the cirrhotic stage (see **Fig. 2**C).

HISTOPATHOLOGY OF ACUTE ALCOHOL-RELATED LIVER DISEASES

In addition to predisposing to development of chronic liver disease, long-term heavy drinking can cause alcohol-related hepatitis (AH), formerly known as alcoholic hepatitis, a clinical syndrome defined by the rapid onset of jaundice, hepatomegaly, elevated liver enzymes, and liver failure in a previously asymptomatic person.[2] AH was once considered synonymous with alcohol-related steatohepatitis (ASH), formerly known as alcoholic steatohepatitis, but there has been recent recognition that terminology should distinguish between the clinical syndrome and the histologic findings. The distinction is necessary because ASH can be found in asymptomatic patients with only mildly deranged liver chemistry and also because the clinical syndrome of AH is sometimes caused by noninflammatory histologic variants of acute ALD (**Table 1**).[3] Each of these patterns of acute liver injury can occur in patients with or without underlying alcohol-related cirrhosis.

Alcohol-Related Steatohepatitis

In contrast to simple steatosis, steatohepatitis is defined by the presence of both hepatocyte injury and inflammation. The predominant mode of cellular injury in ASH is ballooning degeneration of hepatocytes due to a combination of cytoskeletal damage and oncotic swelling, eventually leading to hepatocyte necrosis. Hepatocyte apoptosis may also occur. Ballooned hepatocytes are enlarged, are round, and have cleared and reticulated cytoplasm, with persistence of the centrally placed nuclei. Many ballooned hepatocytes contain ropey, eosinophilic, cytoplasmic inclusions, known as Mallory-Denk bodies, sometimes forming a ring around the nucleus (**Fig. 3**A). The mechanisms leading to Mallory-Denk body formation are an area of active research and beyond the scope of this review. Immunohistochemical staining for the major protein constituents of Mallory-Denk bodies (namely, cytokeratins 8

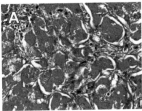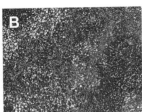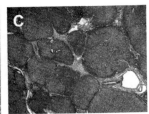

Fig. 2. Progression of fibrosis in ALD (trichrome stain, magnification ×40). (*A*) Use of trichrome stain highlights the bright blue arachnoid or chicken-wire pattern of fine collagen deposition around each hepatocyte. (*B*) Bridging fibrosis links adjacent central veins and adjacent portal tracts and links between centrilobular and periportal zones. (*C*) In alcoholic cirrhosis, complete fibrous septa enclose regenerative nodules.

Table 1
Characteristic histologic features of alcohol-related patterns of liver injury that can cause the clinical syndrome of alcohol-related hepatitis

Histologic Feature	Alcohol-Related Steatohepatitis	Alcohol-Related Foamy Degeneration	Alcohol-related Fatty Liver with Cholestasis
Macrovesicular steatosis	+	−	++
Microvesicular steatosis	+/−	++	−
Hepatocyte ballooning	++	−	−
Mallory-Denk bodies	++	−	−
Inflammation	++	−	−
Fibrosis	+, often ++	+/−	+/−

The relative proportions of histologic findings are given as ++, prominent, +, present, −, absent or minimal, and +/−, variable.

and 18, ubiquitin, and p62), however, can help in their histologic identification. Immunohistochemical staining for cytokeratins 8 and 18 can also help identify ballooned hepatocytes, which have absent or decreased cytoplasmic staining. Lobular inflammation in ASH is typically rich in neutrophils, and the neutrophils may surround ballooned hepatocytes (termed, *satellitosis* [see **Fig. 3A**]). Portal inflammation is usually milder than that seen in other forms of chronic hepatitis, such as viral hepatitis, and may contain a mix of lymphocytes, neutrophils, and even plasma cells, eosinophils, and mast cells. Steatosis (most often macrovesicular or mixed type but sometimes with foci of microvesicular steatosis) is almost always present in ASH, though to variable degrees and not a requisite to a diagnosis of ASH. Likewise, chicken-wire collagen deposition around the ballooned hepatocytes is usually prominent, and portal and periportal fibrosis is often advanced, with a majority of biopsied patients with ASH also having evidence of underlying cirrhosis. In some cases of significant necrosis and dropout of centrilobular hepatocytes, thick confluent fibrosis develops that can completely occlude the central veins, leading to a severe variant of ASH termed, *sclerosing hyaline necrosis*.[4] Other histologic features described in ASH include enlarged

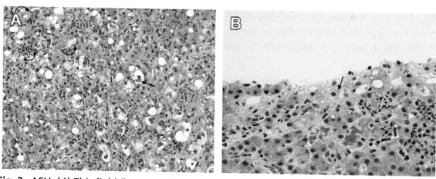

Fig. 3. ASH. (*A*) This field (hematoxylin-eosin stain, magnification ×20) shows ballooned hepatocytes, many of which contain Mallory-Denk bodies (*straight arrow*) as well as lobular inflammation. Satellitosis is present, with neutrophils surrounding and even infiltrating some of the ballooned hepatocytes (*curved arrows*). (*B*) A tiny megamitochondrion (*arrow*) appears as distinct, round, and brighter pink within the wispy cytoplasm of a ballooned hepatocyte (hematoxylin-eosin stain, magnification ×40).

mitochondria (termed, *megamitochondria* [see **Fig. 3**B]), ductular reaction, and perivenular cholestasis.

Alcohol-Related Foamy Degeneration

Alcohol-related foamy degeneration (AFD), formerly known as alcoholic foamy degeneration, is a variant of acute ALD that can cause the clinical syndrome of AH and that is defined by the presence of abundant microvesicular (or small droplet), foamy-appearing steatosis involving the centrilobular and sometimes midzonal hepatocytes (**Fig. 4**). The nuclei of affected hepatocytes remain centrally located. A minor component of macrovesicular fat can be present in some non–zone 3 hepatocytes but is not a prominent feature of this disease. Variable degrees of portal fibrosis, periportal sinusoidal collagen deposition, megamitochondria, and lobular cholestasis can be seen, but, unlike in ASH, ballooned hepatocytes and Mallory-Denk bodies are rare or absent and the degree of lobular and portal inflammation is minimal and composed of mononuclear cells. Consistent with the lack of necroinflammation seen histologically, the pathogenesis of AFD seems degenerative rather than inflammatory. Multiple hepatic mitochondrial DNA deletions have been correlated with AFD.[5,6] Affected hepatocytes have damage to or loss of mitochondria and endoplasmic reticulum seen on electron microscopy and decreased functional activity by enzyme histochemical staining.[7]

Uchida and colleagues[7] first described AFD in a case series of 21 patients biopsied due to ALD at Rancho Los Amigos Hospital in Southern California in 1980. The patients were predominantly male (with a male-to-female ratio of 2.5:1) with a mean age of 42 years (range 26–60 years). All had a long history of heavy alcohol use, with consumption of at least 175 g of ethanol per day. The presenting symptoms and signs were similar to those of patients with ASH and included jaundice (90%) and hepatomegaly (90%). AFD has since been described in multiple other case reports and series from Japan,[8–10] France,[5,6,11] Spain,[12–14] Albania,[15] and the United States.[16,17] The reported prevalence of AFD is 0.8% to 14% among patients biopsied due to ALD. Despite associated with the clinical syndrome of AH, many of the reported cases of AFD had clinical recovery within weeks of alcohol abstinence and supportive care. Similarly, an autopsy study, discussed briefly in Uchida and

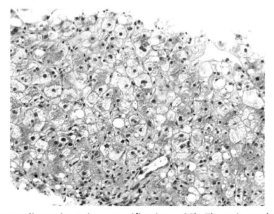

Fig. 4. AFD (hematoxylin-eosin stain, magnification ×20). There is marked microvesicular steatosis with hepatocytes containing abundant small fat droplets. The hepatocytes are enlarged by fat droplets but their nuclei remain centrally placed, making them appear similar to ballooned hepatocytes to an untrained eye. No Mallory-Denk bodies are seen and lobular inflammation is minimal.

colleaguess'[7] original publication, noted that among 124 patients who died of liver-related complications at their center in 1979 to 1980, 35% had ASH whereas only 4% had striking AFD without ASH. On the other hand, AFD was fatal in a third of the patients describe in a small French series.[6] To date, no specific treatment of AFD has been proposed.

Alcohol-Related Fatty Liver with Cholestasis

Alcohol-related fatty liver with cholestasis (AFLC) is another variant of acute ALD that can cause the clinical syndrome of AH or that can mimic the clinical presentation of obstructive jaundice. Unlike AFD, AFLC is defined by abundant macrovesicular, not microvesicular, steatosis (**Fig. 5**). Cholestasis is often present (see **Fig. 5**), but the degree of portal fibrosis is variable, ranging from minimal fibrosis to underlying cirrhosis. Similar to AFD and in contrast to ASH, ballooned hepatocytes and Mallory-Denk bodies are absent and portal and lobular inflammation is mild. Until recently, evidence of AFLC was mainly limited to a few older case series describing noncirrhotic patients.[18–21] Multiple patients with AFLC, however, either with or without cirrhosis were identified in a recent retrospective study of 172 patients biopsied due to the clinical syndrome of severe AH.[17] The mechanism of cholestasis that occurs in AFLC is not yet established.

PEARLS AND PITFALLS OF LIVER BIOPSY IN THE DIAGNOSIS AND MANAGEMENT OF ALCOHOL-RELATED LIVER DISEASES
What Other Diseases Can Have Histopathology Similar to Alcohol-Related Liver Diseases?

The histologic features typically found in ALD are not unique to an alcohol-related liver injury (**Table 2**). Macrovesicular steatosis is a common histologic finding in patients without any significant alcohol history, especially among those who are obese.[22] Obesity and other components of the metabolic syndrome including diabetes also predispose to development of nonalcoholic steatohepatitis (NASH) that can lead to cirrhosis.[22] Less commonly, macrovesicular steatosis and steatohepatitis with hepatocyte ballooning and Mallory-Denk bodies can be caused by Wilson disease[23] or

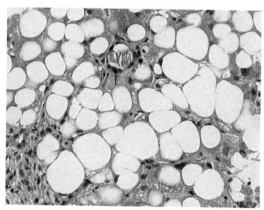

Fig. 5. AFLC (hematoxylin-eosin stain, magnification ×40). There is marked macrovesicular steatosis, with hepatocytes containing large fat droplets that displace the nuclei to the periphery of the cells. Marked cholestasis, including a canalicular bile plug (*arrow*) is seen but no lobular inflammation, ballooned hepatocytes, or Mallory-Denk bodies.

| | Macrovesicular | |
Macrovesicular Steatosis	Steatohepatitis	Microvesicular Steatosis
Alcohol-related steatosis	ASH	AFD
NAFLD	Nonalcoholic	Acute fatty liver of pregnancy
Wilson disease	steatohepatitis	Vinyl chloride
Total parenteral nutrition	Wilson disease	Drug-induced: aspirin (Reye
Drug-induced: glucocorticoids,	Drug-induced:	syndrome), tetracycline, valproic
amiodarone, chemotherapy	amiodarone,	acid, cocaine, nonsteroidal anti-
(eg, methotrexate, tamoxifen,	chemotherapy	inflammatory drugs (eg,
irinotecan, 5-fluorouracil,	(eg, methotrexate,	ibuprofen and naproxen),
cisplatin, and asparaginase)	tamoxifen, and	nucleoside reverse transcriptase
	irinotecan)	inhibitors (eg, zidovudine and
		didanosine)

Table 2
Differential diagnosis for histologic patterns of alcohol-related liver injury

certain drugs,[24] such as amiodarone,[25] tamoxifen,[26] methotrexate,[27] or irinotecan.[28] It is important to consider these possibilities in the differential diagnosis for patients with histologic steatohepatitis, even in those who drink alcohol or are obese with metabolic risk factors, because drug cessation or treatment of copper accumulation in affected patients can reverse steatohepatitis and prevent fibrosis progression. Drug-induced liver injury should also be considered in patients with pure microvesicular steatosis, because the histology of AFD is similar to that seen in other conditions associated with abnormal mitochondrial fatty acid oxidation, including Reye syndrome and liver injury caused by tetracycline, valproic acid, nonsteroidal anti-inflammatory drugs (ibuprofen and naproxen), nucleoside reverse transcriptase inhibitors (zidovudine and didanosine), and cocaine.[24] Acute fatty liver of pregnancy is a rare but serious condition occurring in the third trimester of pregnancy that is also characterized by very fine, small-droplet steatosis on histology.[29] Sclerosing hyaline necrosis is the only pattern of liver injury that may be almost pathognomonic to ALD, although there is 1 case report in the literature of sclerosing hyaline necrosis and Mallory-Denk bodies found on intraoperative liver biopsy performed in a 37-year-old man with no reported history of alcohol consumption and with Bloom syndrome, an extremely rare autosomal recessive genetic disorder.[30]

What Histologic Clues Can Help Differentiate Between Alcohol-Related and Nonalcoholic Fatty Liver Disease?

On the basis of histology alone, nonalcoholic fatty liver disease (NAFLD) may be indistinguishable from ALD, and it is usually impossible to prove the presence of ALD based on liver biopsy in a patient with no significant self-reported alcohol history. In such cases, collateral history obtained from a patient's family, friends, and other treating medical practitioners is often more valuable than a liver biopsy. A model based on patients' gender, body mass index, ratio of aspartate aminotransferase (AST) to alanine aminotransferase (ALT), and mean corpuscular volume may also help discriminate between ASH and NASH in patients with an unreliable alcohol history.[31] Many patients who chronically consume excessive amounts of alcohol, however, also have comorbid risk factors for NAFLD, and their liver disease can be due to overlapping injury from both conditions. That said, NAFLD does not usually present acutely with a clinical syndrome like AH, except perhaps in some cases of acute-on-chronic liver failure triggered by sepsis or gastrointestinal hemorrhage in patients with previously undiagnosed and well-compensated NASH cirrhosis.[32,33]

In patients in whom a drug-induced liver injury has been excluded, 2 histologic patterns of liver injury—pure microvesicular steatosis and sclerosing hyaline necrosis—can confidently distinguish ALD from NAFLD because they do not occur with NAFLD. Other histologic features of ASH overlap with those seen in NASH but may differ in degrees (**Table 3**). Portal inflammation is more common and of higher grade in ASH than NASH. The predominant inflammatory cells are also different in the 2 conditions, typically neutrophils in ASH but lymphocytes in NASH. Mallory-Denk bodies are more frequent and may be larger and coarser in ASH, whereas acidophil bodies (also known as Councilman bodies) from apoptosis are seen more frequently in NASH. The degree of macrovesicular steatosis is variable in ASH but typically remains high in NASH. Advanced hepatic fibrosis can accompany both conditions, but thick fibrous scars are suggestive of an alcohol-associated liver injury. Marked cholestasis is usually due to acute decompensation and is uncommon in patients with NASH.

Are There Histologic Clues That Can Help Determine How Recently a Patient Has Been Drinking Alcohol?

With abstinence from alcohol, steatosis usually disappears within 6 weeks to 8 weeks, although large fat droplets that have a high surface-to-volume ratio are less susceptible to the action of lipases and can persist for a few months after cessation of drinking. Macrovesicular steatosis can also remain prevalent in patients who cease drinking but have obesity or other metabolic risk factors predisposing to nonalcoholic fatty liver. The histologic features of ASH typically resolve within 4 months to 6 months of alcohol cessation, first with resolution of neutrophilic infiltrates, followed by disappearance of megamitochondria, Mallory-Denk bodies, and hepatocyte ballooning. Pericellular fibrosis regresses with abstinence, and fibrous septa become thinner. In patients with cirrhosis who are actively drinking, the regenerative cirrhotic nodules tend to be smaller (micronodular cirrhosis), whereas the nodules become larger and well demarcated (macronodular cirrhosis) in patients who remain abstinent.[34]

Is a Liver Biopsy Necessary to Diagnose and Manage Alcohol-Related Hepatitis?

The question of whether or not to perform a liver biopsy in a patient with the clinical syndrome of AH is controversial. Although the clinical syndrome of AH is most closely

Table 3
Characteristic histologic features of alcohol-related steatohepatitis versus nonalcoholic steatohepatitis

Histologic Feature	Alcohol-Related Steatohepatitis	Nonalcoholic Steatohepatitis
Macrovesicular steatosis	+	++
Microvesicular steatosis	+/−	+/−
Hepatocyte ballooning	++	+
Mallory-Denk bodies	++	+/−
Neutrophilic inflammation	++	+
Pericellular fibrosis	++	+
Central hyaline sclerosis	+/−	−
Portal fibrosis	+, often ++	+/−
Cholestasis	+	+/−

The relative proportions of histologic findings are given as ++, prominent, +, present, −, absent or minimal, and +/−, variable.

associated with ASH, other liver diseases, including ischemic hepatitis, drug-induced liver injury, autoimmune hepatitis, viral hepatitis, and biliary obstruction, can mimic it. Even if non–alcohol-related causes of jaundice are excluded, AH can be caused by sepsis in patients with alcohol-related cirrhosis or by noninflammatory variants of acute ALD (in particular, AFD and AFLC).[3] A crucial point of contention among experts is how often AH occurs without histologic ASH. A second point of contention is whether certain clinical and laboratory parameters can discriminate between patients with and without ASH.

One prior study found that almost half of patients with acute decompensation of ALD did not have histologic ASH.[35] Two more recent studies among patients with clinical AH that were not specifically designed to address the question of diagnostic accuracy also reported that greater than 35% of the patients biopsied did not have ASH.[14,36] Other studies suggest that the proportion of patients with AH who lack ASH is likely more modest, in the range of 4% to 26%,[17,37–40] especially if biopsy is limited to patients with severe AH with a total bilirubin level of at least 5 mg/dL and Maddrey discriminant function of at least 32.[17,37,38,40] Leukocytosis in patients with AH and without active infection has been reported to have a very high positive predictive value for histologic ASH.[17,38] Although some experts[41] and recently published clinical practice guidelines[42] suggest that a probable clinical diagnosis of ASH also requires an ALT level less than 400 IU/L and a ratio of AST to ALT of at least 1.5, those criteria have not yet been demonstrated to accurately discriminate between patients with and without histologic ASH on biopsy.

In centers where transjugular liver biopsy is available, the costs and risks of performing and interpreting a biopsy need to be carefully weighed against the potential harms of making an incorrect diagnosis based on physicians' clinical impressions alone. If corticosteroids or an investigational therapy is contemplated, then liver biopsy should be considered, especially in patients without leukocytosis. Corticosteroids, which currently remain the mainstay of pharmaceutical therapy for severe ASH, are not indicated and may even be harmful for patients without histologic ASH. Similarly, many of the therapies currently under investigation for treatment of ASH target cellular pathways—such as apoptosis or activation of the innate immune system—that may not play a role in the pathogenesis of AFD or AFLC. For clinical trials, immunohistochemical data obtained from patients' liver biopsies may also provide important insights leading to new therapeutic strategies.[43]

In contrast, if no medical treatment of AH is planned, then biopsy is rarely necessary unless for the purpose of diagnosing a non–alcohol-related disease, such as an autoimmune hepatitis or a drug-induced liver injury. In patients with AH but with an uncertain alcohol history, biopsy has been used to help ascertain the diagnosis[42] and can have implications on patients' candidacy for liver transplantation. Given the histologic similarities between ASH and NASH, as discussed previously, however, the authors recommend caution with biopsy for that purpose alone, especially in patients with metabolic risk factors. Performing a liver biopsy also does not influence the likelihood of patients' maintaining long-term abstinence from alcohol.[44] There is a validated prognostic scoring system based on histologic features for patients with ASH,[39] but performing biopsy for prognostication is not recommended in routine clinical practice given the availability of multiple other well-validated AH prognostic scoring systems based on static and dynamic noninvasive laboratory parameters.[45]

How Reliable Is Liver Biopsy in the Diagnosis of Alcohol-Related Liver Diseases?

The diagnostic performance of liver biopsy depends on (1) accurate and reproducible interpretation of the histology by an experienced pathologist and (2) a basic assumption that the minute amount of tissue collected through a biopsy has histology that is representative of the entire liver parenchyma. The former issue is addressed by assessing observer variation (or, conversely, interobserver agreement) for histology whereas the latter issue is addressed by assessing for sampling variability of biopsy. Liver biopsy in the diagnosis of ALD is imperfect but satisfactory in both regards.

In the largest study on observer variation in diagnosis of ALD, 2 experienced liver pathologists independently assessed 362 biopsies from patients with heavy alcohol consumption on 41 histologic features.[46] Interobserver agreement was excellent for cirrhosis ($\kappa = 0.84$), moderate for key features of ASH, including hepatocyte ballooning ($\kappa = 0.47$), Mallory-Denk bodies ($\kappa = 0.50$), and lobular inflammation ($\kappa = 0.54$), and fair for the degree of steatosis ($\kappa = 0.35$).[46] Similar interobserver agreement has been reported for features of NASH, although with higher interobserver agreement for the degree of steatosis ($\kappa = 0.79$).[47] Worse, but still overall satisfactory, interobserver agreement for the main diagnostic features of ASH was reported in smaller, recent studies.[17,48] Ensuring an adequately sized liver biopsy (ideally, at least 2–3 cm in length and 16-gauge in caliber, with at least 11 complete portal tracts) improves the accuracy and reproducibility of histologic interpretation.[1,49] For patients with suspected ASH, histologic interpretation may also be improved with immunohistochemical stains for keratins 8 and 18 for hepatocyte ballooning[35] and ubiquitin for Mallory-Denk bodies[50] or use of digital morphometrics,[17,51] although these methods are not necessary in routine clinical practice.

Because the liver is not homogeneous and a typical liver biopsy specimen represents only approximately 1/50,000 of the total mass of the liver, sampling variability is a concern.[52] Two early studies using repeated punctures of the liver reported little to no sampling discordance for ASH but included few patients with that diagnosis.[53,54] More recent studies have addressed the issue of sampling variability for patients with NASH. In a study of 51 patients with NAFLD who each underwent percutaneous biopsy of the right hepatic lobe with 2 passes, sampling agreement was good for steatosis grade ($\kappa = 0.64$) and moderate for fibrosis stage ($\kappa = 0.47$) and hepatocyte ballooning ($\kappa = 0.45$) but fair-to-poor for Mallory-Denk bodies ($\kappa = 0.27$) and lobular inflammation ($\kappa = 0.13$).[55] A study conducted among 58 patients who each underwent 2 intraoperative biopsies of the left hepatic lobe during laparoscopic Roux-en-Y gastric bypass surgery showed excellent sampling agreement for presence or absence of steatosis or zone 3 ballooning and moderate sampling agreement for presence of portal fibrosis,[56] but the study did not include any patients with advanced fibrosis and did not assess sampling variability for lobular inflammation or Mallory-Denk bodies. Both studies were limited to paired biopsies taken from the sample lobe of the liver. Paired right and left hepatic lobe biopsies taken intraoperatively during open Roux-en-Y gastric bypass surgery among 10 patients showed no discordances in steatohepatitis grade but 30% discordance in fibrosis stage.[57] Whether these results apply to patients with steatohepatitis related to alcohol is uncertain. New studies addressing sampling variability in patients with ALD are difficult to design because of ethical concerns with performing multiple biopsies. It is possible that explant data from patients who undergo liver transplantation due to ALD can yield additional information.

SUMMARY

Liver biopsy is not necessary for diagnosis of most patients with ALD, such as those with simple steatosis or alcohol-related cirrhosis. Due to the overlap between features of ASH and NASH, biopsy is not recommended to ascertain a diagnosis of ALD in patients with an uncertain alcohol history unless the clinical syndrome of AH is present. In patients with the clinical syndrome of AH with rapid onset of jaundice and liver failure, liver biopsy remains the gold standard for distinguishing between steatohepatitis that may benefit from corticosteroids or investigational drugs and noninflammatory histologic patterns of injury, such as AFD and AFLC, that do not have any approved or investigational pharmacologic therapies.

ACKNOWLEDGMENTS

The authors would like to acknowledge the Division of Liver Diseases and the Department of Pathology at The Mount Sinai Hospital for their academic and funding support during the preparation of this manuscript.

REFERENCES

1. Rockey DC, Caldwell SH, Goodman ZD, et al. American Association for the study of liver diseases. Liver biopsy. Hepatology 2009;49(3):1017–44.
2. Chayanupatkul M, Liangpunsakul S. Alcoholic hepatitis: a comprehensive review of pathogenesis and treatment. World J Gastroenterol 2014;20(20):6279–86.
3. Roth N, Kanel G, Kaplowitz N. Alcoholic foamy degeneration and alcoholic fatty liver with jaundice: often overlooked causes of jaundice and hepatic decompensation that can mimic alcoholic hepatitis. Clin Liver Dis 2016;6(6):145–8.
4. Goodman ZD, Ishak KG. Occlusive venous lesions in alcoholic liver disease. A study of 200 cases. Gastroenterology 1982;83(4):786–96.
5. Fromenty B, Grimbert S, Mansouri A, et al. Hepatic mitochondrial DNA deletion in alcoholics: association with microvesicular steatosis. Gastroenterology 1995; 108(1):193–200.
6. Mansouri A, Fromenty B, Berson A, et al. Multiple hepatic mitochondrial DNA deletions suggest premature oxidative aging in alcoholic patients. J Hepatol 1997; 27(1):96–102.
7. Uchida T, Kao H, Quispe-Sjogren M, et al. Alcoholic foamy degeneration–a pattern of acute alcoholic injury of the liver. Gastroenterology 1983;84(4):683–92.
8. Koyama W, Kanayama M, Uchida T, et al. Alcoholic foamy degeneration. Kanzo 1984;25(5):657–65.
9. Uchida T, Shikata T, Govindarajan S, et al. The characteristics of alcoholic liver disease in Japan. Clinicopathologic comparison with alcoholic liver disease in the United States. Liver 1987;7(5):290–7.
10. Shiomi S, Sasaki N, Yokogawa T, et al. Usefulness of scintigraphy with Tc-99m phytate for the diagnosis of alcoholic foamy degeneration. Clin Nucl Med 1998; 23(5):302–4.
11. Fléjou JF, Degott C, Kharsa G, et al. Alcoholic foamy steatosis: study of 3 cases. Gastroenterol Clin Biol 1987;11(2):165–8 [in French].
12. Montull S, Parés A, Bruguera M, et al. Alcoholic foamy degeneration in Spain. Prevalence and clinico-pathological features. Liver 1989;9(2):79–85.
13. Ruiz P, Michelena J, Altamirano J, et al. Hepatic hemodynamics and transient elastography in alcoholic foamy degeneration: report of 2 cases. Ann Hepatol 2012;11(3):399–403.
14. Bissonnette J, Altamirano J, Devue C, et al. A Prospective study of the utility of plasma biomarkers to diagnose alcoholic hepatitis. Hepatology 2017. https://doi.org/10.1002/hep.29080.
15. Kondili LA, Taliani G, Cerga G, et al. Correlation of alcohol consumption with liver histological features in non-cirrhotic patients. Eur J Gastroenterol Hepatol 2005; 17(2):155–9.

16. Suri S, Mitros FA, Ahluwalia JP. Alcoholic foamy degeneration and a markedly elevated GGT: a case report and literature review. Dig Dis Sci 2003;48(6):1142–6.

17. Roth NC, Saberi B, Macklin J, et al. Prediction of histologic alcoholic hepatitis based on clinical presentation limits the need for liver biopsy. Hepatol Commun 2017;1(10):1070–84.

18. Zieve L. Jaundice, hyperlipemia and hemolytic anemia: a heretofore unrecognized syndrome associated with alcoholic fatty liver and cirrhosis. Ann Intern Med 1958;48(3):471–96.

19. Ballard H, Bernstein M, Farrar JT. Fatty liver presenting as obstructive jaundice. Am J Med 1961;30:196–201.

20. Sataline LR, Matre WJ. Significance of hyperphosphatasemia in alcoholics with liver disease. an analysis of fifty-eight cases, with histologic diagnoses. Am J Med 1963;35:323–42.

21. Morgan MY, Sherlock S, Scheuer PJ. Acute cholestasis, hepatic failure, and fatty liver in the alcoholic. Scand J Gastroenterol 1978;13(3):299–303.

22. Wanless IR, Lentz JS. Fatty liver hepatitis (steatohepatitis) and obesity: an autopsy study with analysis of risk factors. Hepatology 1990;12(5):1106–10.

23. Mahmood S, Inada N, Izumi A, et al. Wilson's disease masquerading as nonalcoholic steatohepatitis. N Am J Med Sci 2009;1(2):74–6.

24. Patel V, Sanyal AJ. Drug-induced steatohepatitis. Clin Liver Dis 2013;17(4):533–46.

25. Raja K, Thung SN, Fiel MI, et al. Drug-induced steatohepatitis leading to cirrhosis: long-term toxicity of amiodarone use. Semin Liver Dis 2009;29(4):423–8.

26. Saphner T, Triest-Robertson S. Non-alcoholic steatohepatitis (NASH) in patients with breast cancer and association with tamoxifen. J Clin Oncol 2008;26(15_suppl):11528.

27. Amacher DE, Chalasani N. Drug-induced hepatic steatosis. Semin Liver Dis 2014;34(2):205–14.

28. Yahagi M, Tsuruta M, Hasegawa H, et al. Non-alcoholic fatty liver disease fibrosis score predicts hematological toxicity of chemotherapy including irinotecan for colorectal cancer. Mol Clin Oncol 2017;6(4):529–33.

29. Rolfes DB, Ishak KG. Acute fatty liver of pregnancy: a clinicopathologic study of 35 cases. Hepatology 1985;5(6):1149–58.

30. Wang J, Cornford ME, German J, et al. Sclerosing hyaline necrosis of the liver in Bloom syndrome. Arch Pathol Lab Med 1999;123(4):346–50.

31. Dunn W, Angulo P, Sanderson S, et al. Utility of a new model to diagnose an alcohol basis for steatohepatitis. Gastroenterology 2006;131(4):1057–63.

32. Hernaez R, Solà E, Moreau R, et al. Acute-on-chronic liver failure: an update. Gut 2017;66(3):541–53.

33. Blasco-Algora S, Masegosa-Ataz J, Gutiérrez-García ML, et al. Acute-on-chronic liver failure: pathogenesis, prognostic factors and management. World J Gastroenterol 2015;21(42):12125–40.

34. Kanel GC, Korula J. Atlas of liver pathology. 3rd edition. Philadelphia: Saunders Elsevier; 2011.

35. Mookerjee RP, Lackner C, Stauber R, et al. The role of liver biopsy in the diagnosis and prognosis of patients with acute deterioration of alcoholic cirrhosis. J Hepatol 2011;55(5):1103–11.

36. Lackner C, Spindelboeck W, Haybaeck J, et al. Histological parameters and alcohol abstinence determine long-term prognosis in patients with alcoholic liver disease. J Hepatol 2017;66(3):610–8.

37. Hamid R, Forrest EH. Is histology required for the diagnosis of alcoholic hepatitis? A review of published randomised controlled trials. Gut 2011;60(Suppl 1):A233.
38. Hardy T, Wells C, Kendrick S, et al. White cell count and platelet count associate with histological alcoholic hepatitis in jaundiced harmful drinkers. BMC Gastroenterol 2013;13(1):55.
39. Altamirano J, Miquel R, Katoonizadeh A, et al. A histologic scoring system for prognosis of patients with alcoholic hepatitis. Gastroenterology 2014;146(5): 1231–9.e1–6.
40. Petts G, Lloyd K, Vergis N, et al. PWE-113 the liver biopsy in alcoholic hepatitis: data from the steroids or pentoxifylline in alcoholic hepatitis (stopah) clinical trial. Gut 2015;64(Suppl 1). A262.
41. Crabb DW, Bataller R, Chalasani NP, et al. Standard definitions and common data elements for clinical trials in patients with alcoholic hepatitis: recommendation from the NIAAA alcoholic hepatitis consortia. Gastroenterology 2016;150:785–90.
42. Singal AK, Bataller R, Ahn J, et al. ACG clinical guideline: alcoholic liver disease. Am J Gastroenterol 2018;113(2):175–94.
43. Lieber SR, Rice JP, Lucey MR, et al. Controversies in clinical trials for alcoholic hepatitis. J Hepatol 2018;68(3):586–92.
44. Trabut J-B, Plat A, Thepot V, et al. Influence of liver biopsy on abstinence in alcohol-dependent patients. Alcohol Alcohol 2008;43(5):559–63.
45. Louvet A, Labreuche J, Artru F, et al. Combining data from liver disease scoring systems better predicts outcomes of patients with alcoholic hepatitis. Gastroenterology 2015;149(2):398–406.e8 [quiz: e16–7].
46. Bedossa P, Poynard T, Naveau S, et al. Observer variation in assessment of liver biopsies of alcoholic patients. Alcohol Clin Exp Res 1988;12(1):173–8.
47. Kleiner DE, Brunt EM, Van Natta M, et al. Design and validation of a histological scoring system for nonalcoholic fatty liver disease. Hepatology 2005;41(6):1313–21.
48. Horvath B, Allende D, Xie H, et al. Interobserver variability in scoring liver biopsies with a diagnosis of alcoholic hepatitis. Alcohol Clin Exp Res 2017;41(9):1568–73.
49. Kalambokis G, Manousou P, Vibhakorn S, et al. Transjugular liver biopsy–indications, adequacy, quality of specimens, and complications–a systematic review. J Hepatol 2007;47(2):284–94.
50. Vyberg M, Leth P. Ubiquitin: an immunohistochemical marker of Mallory bodies and alcoholic liver disease. APMIS Suppl 1991;23:46–52.
51. Vanderbeck S, Bockhorst J, Kleiner D, et al. Automatic quantification of lobular inflammation and hepatocyte ballooning in nonalcoholic fatty liver disease liver biopsies. Hum Pathol 2015;46(5):767–75.
52. Bravo AA, Sheth SG, Chopra S. Liver biopsy. N Engl J Med 2001;344(7):495–500.
53. Baunsgaard P, Sanchez GC, Lundborg CJ. The variation of pathological changes in the liver evaluated by double biopsies. Acta Pathol Microbiol Scand A 1979; 87(1):51–7.
54. Abdi W, Millan JC, Mezey E. Sampling variability on percutaneous liver biopsy. Arch Intern Med 1979;139(6):667–9.
55. Ratziu V, Charlotte F, Heurtier A, et al. Sampling variability of liver biopsy in nonalcoholic fatty liver disease. Gastroenterology 2005;128(7):1898–906.
56. Arun J, Jhala N, Lazenby AJ, et al. Influence of liver biopsy heterogeneity and diagnosis of nonalcoholic steatohepatitis in subjects undergoing gastric bypass. Obes Surg 2007;17(2):155–61.
57. Janiec DJ, Jacobson ER, Freeth A, et al. Histologic variation of grade and stage of non-alcoholic fatty liver disease in liver biopsies. Obes Surg 2005;15(4): 497–501.

Alcohol and the Law

Maya Balakrishnan, MD, MPH*, Stephen Chris Pappas, MD, JD[1]

KEYWORDS

- Alcohol • Law • Public safety • Alcohol-related impairment • Patient confidentiality

KEY POINTS

- It is important for physicians to be aware of the local procedures for reporting alcohol use and related impairment and to have some knowledge of the law applicable in the jurisdiction where they practice.
- The physician's duty is patient education with an ethical and legal duty to warn the patient of the adverse personal and societal effects of alcohol. If possible, family support should be enlisted and alcohol rehabilitation efforts pursued.
- The physician should explicitly document all good faith efforts to accomplish these initiatives.
- Warning third parties of the potential for harm related to an individual patient's alcohol-related impairment may involve a breach of patient confidentiality.
- Disclosure to a third party should be undertaken only if the risk of significant harm exceeds the burden that will result to the patient from warning others. Although specific laws, guidelines, and provider protections exist, in general, the law remains vague in this area.

Alcohol has been ubiquitous throughout history. Despite widespread knowledge of its adverse medical and social effects and laws regulating its use, it remains the most widely available abused psychoactive substance in the world. Beyond the immediate medical consequences of alcohol abuse, the link with criminal acts such as traffic accidents and fatalities, crimes (particularly murder, rape, and assault), child abuse, and domestic violence results in alcohol placing tremendous economic and social burdens on society.[1] Clinicians taking care of patients with alcohol-related liver disease will encounter instances in which their medical, ethical, legal, and public health responsibilities intersect and may conflict. This article explores some basic medical concepts relevant to legal proceedings, the assessment of acute and recent alcohol use and impairment and the use of those assessments, and a clarification of a physician's

Disclosure Statement: The authors have nothing to disclose.
Section of Gastroenterology, Department of Medicine, Baylor College of Medicine, 1 Baylor Plaza, Houston, TX 77030, USA
[1] Present address: 34 Glowing Star Place, The Woodlands, TX 77382.
* Corresponding author. Ben Taub General Hospital, 5th Floor, Office 5 PO 71-006, 1504 Taub Loop, Houston, TX 77030.
E-mail address: Maya.balakrishnan@bcm.edu

Clin Liver Dis 23 (2019) 25–38
https://doi.org/10.1016/j.cld.2018.09.002
1089-3261/19/© 2018 Elsevier Inc. All rights reserved.

duty to warn in the contexts of acute alcohol ingestion, alcoholic cirrhosis, and hepatic encephalopathy (HE).

SOME BASIC FACTS USEFUL FOR LAW ENFORCEMENT AND LEGAL CONSIDERATIONS

The majority of alcohol-related law enforcement proceedings revolve around acute intoxication. As such, it is useful to review some basic facts that law enforcement officers will often take into account when establishing whether someone may be alcohol impaired, and on which a physician may be asked to comment, either in an expert testimony setting or when looking after a patient in police custody. The rule of thumb for what constitutes a drink seems to start with any beverage that contains approximately 14 to 15 g of pure alcohol.[2] This translates into 10 to 12 ounces of beer, 5 to 6 ounces of wine, and 1.5 ounces (45 mL) of hard spirits. The blood alcohol concentration (BAC) can be roughly estimated assuming 1 drink will produce a BAC of 0.02% for a 200-pound male and 0.04% for a 125-pound female.[3] The time to peak BAC after ingestion of alcohol varies widely, from approximately 40 minutes on an empty stomach to approximately 15 minutes when food has been ingested.[3] Although BAC correlates with manifestations of intoxication, the degree varies widely between individuals. It is therefore important to distinguish between having a BAC above an allowable legal limit and being impaired. These facts are useful for law enforcement to initially roughly assess whether someone in their custody has consumed enough alcohol to raise their BAC above the legal limit (to be confirmed by measuring BAC), or to be impaired (also to be confirmed by testing and testimony). BAC is most important for criminal laws establishing statutory BAC limits for driving, currently a BAC of 0.08% in most American jurisdictions.[3] Intoxication is relevant to criminal liability associated with alcohol intake and impairment and voluntary and involuntary intoxication. For some crimes requiring an element of a specific mental state or intent (eg, burglary), voluntary intoxication may serve as a defense.

Although law enforcement is most commonly involved with the assessment of acute alcohol intoxication, the physician is far more likely to be required to assess recent ongoing alcohol use and, occasionally, acute alcohol consumption. It is important to note that although law enforcement, and in some settings, employers, can request alcohol testing and assessment of impairment on the basis of a reasonable suspicion, and subsequently act as dictated by the applicable law, alcohol use and impairment testing by a physician in the office is considered a medical examination. Accordingly, physician-ordered results are subject to all the usual privacy privileges, except in the rare setting when matters are proceeding under a warrant. This factor becomes important regarding what a physician can do with alcohol testing results when they become available, and in particular, the duties to report and duty to warn. This situation is best illustrated by considering the following case scenarios.

ASSESSMENT OF ACUTE AND RECENT ONGOING ALCOHOL USE

A 41-year-old man with compensated cirrhosis related to alcohol presents for follow-up. He lost his driver's license several months ago after a conviction for driving under the influence of alcohol and is participating in a court-ordered rehabilitation program mandating abstinence. During the visit you notice that he is mildly inattentive, slurs his speech, and has a faint smell of alcohol on his breath. He drove himself to the clinic and plans to drive back home afterward. He denies drinking alcohol for the past 2 months and specifically denies that he has had any today. How do you assess and diagnose recent and/or ongoing alcohol use? If you believe your patient is under the influence of alcohol, what is your public responsibility?

There are 3 main categories of testing for alcohol exposure: patient-reported history, indirect alcohol biomarkers, and direct alcohol measurement and biomarkers. Making a choice between methods really depends on the nature of the query at hand (whether recent vs chronic alcohol use; any vs excessive alcohol use), an understanding of the diagnostic limitations of each (confounding factors, duration of detection window), and the need for diagnostic certainty (alcohol screening in the context of possible alcohol related disease vs documentation as part of transplant evaluation). Complete alcohol cessation is imperative to improving survival from alcohol-related liver disease. Thus, clinicians are nearly always interested in confirming that their patients with alcohol-related liver disease have completely ceased all alcohol use. In this patient, there is the additional need to determine whether he has acutely consumed alcohol. This determination could be easily accomplished with breath analysis, the most common practical method used to establish recent acute ingestion, and would be helpful to differentiate alcohol intoxication from HE.

Patient-Reported History

Alcohol use history is most commonly assessed through patient-reported history using tools such as the Alcohol Use Disorders Identification Test (AUDIT; **Table 1**) and the CAGE (**Box 1**). It is important to bear in mind that these really are screening tests designed to detect alcohol dependence or harmful alcohol use (meaning excessive alcohol use at a threshold associated with increased risk for adverse health effects) or alcohol dependence. Alcohol report tools are most useful if positive by ruling in ongoing hazardous alcohol exposure and can aid in diagnosing alcohol-related disease.

The AUDIT, developed and validated by the World Health Organization, is considered the gold standard clinical screen for harmful alcohol use, meaning 21 drinks or more on average per week for men and 14 drinks or more on average per week for women. The short form of the questionnaire, the AUDIT-C, consists of the first 3 questions of the full AUDIT (see **Table 1**). An affirmative response to question 3 indicates excessive alcohol use. An affirmative response should also trigger completion of a full AUDIT questionnaire, where a score of greater than 8 qualifies alcohol use disorder and a score of greater than 20 indicates alcohol dependence.[4,5] The CAGE (see **Box 1**) is a quick screen that specifically detects alcohol dependence with a pooled sensitivity of 0.71 and specificity of 0.90 for a cutoff of 2 or greater.[4] It is not designed to pick up on harmful alcohol use.[6]

These tools, however, rely entirely on patients' candor. Thus, in many high-stakes instances—especially legal concerns, ongoing alcohol rehabilitation, or possible recidivism—there is often a need for objective measures of alcohol intake when patients deny significant alcohol use.

Indirect Biomarkers

Indirect alcohol biomarkers identify alcohol exposure by gauging alcohol's effects on hepatocytes and the metabolism of transferrin and phospholipids. They include alanine aminotransferase, aspartate aminotransferase, gamma glutamyl transferase (GGT), mean corpuscular volume (MCV), carbohydrate-deficient transferrin (CDT), and phosphatidyl ethanol (PEth). With the exception of PEth, this category of biomarkers is best suited to identify chronic excess alcohol exposure (over the course of weeks) and cannot discern recent alcohol use (ongoing for recent days). PEth is the only indirect biomarker that can do so. Finally, the diagnostic accuracy of each

Table 1
Patient self-report tools: AUDIT

Questions	0	1	2	3	4
1. How often do you have a drink containing alcohol?[a]	Never	Monthly or less	2–4 times/mo	2–3 times/wk	>4 times/wk
2. How many drinks containing alcohol do you have on a typical day when you are drinking?[a]	1 or 2	3 or 4	5 or 6	weekly	≥10
3. How often do you have ≥6 drinks on 1 occasion?[a]	Never	Less than monthly	Monthly	Weekly	Daily or almost daily
4. How often in the last year have you found that you were not able to stop drinking once you had started?	Never	Less than monthly	Monthly	Weekly	Daily or almost daily
5. How often in during the last year have you failed to do what was normally expected from you because of drinking?	Never	Less than monthly	Monthly	Weekly	Daily or almost daily
6. How often during the last year have you needed a first drink in the morning to get yourself going after a heavy drinking session?	Never	Less than monthly	Monthly	Weekly	Daily or almost daily
7. How often during the last year have you had a feeling of guilt or remorse after drinking	Never	Less than monthly	Monthly	Weekly	Daily or almost daily
8. How often during the last year have you been unable to remember what happened the night before because you had been drinking?	Never	Less than monthly	Monthly	Weekly	Daily or almost daily
9. Have you or someone else been injured as a result of your drinking?	No		Yes, but not in the last year		Yes, during the last year
10. Has a relative or friend or a doctor or another health worker been concerned about your drinking or suggested you cut down?	No		Yes, but not in the last year		Yes, during the last year

Abbreviation: AUDIT, Alcohol Use Disorders Identification Test.
[a] These 3 questions constitute the AUDIT-C.
Adapted from https://www.drugabuse.gov/sites/default/files/files/AUDIT; with permission. Accessed May 30, 2018.

> **Box 1**
> **Patient self-report tools: CAGE**
>
> 1. Have you ever felt you should Cut down on your drinking?
>
> 2. Have people Annoyed you by criticizing your drinking?
>
> 3. Have you ever felt bad or Guilty about your drinking?
>
> 4. Have you ever had a drink first thing in the morning to steady your nerves or to get rid of a hangover (Eye opener?)
>
> *Adapted from* John A. "Detecting Alcoholism: The CAGE Questionnaire" JAMA 252: 1905-1907; Oct. 12, 1984 [PMID 6471323].

marker is variably influenced by concomitant medical conditions and should be interpreted carefully with this in mind.

Among patients without underlying chronic liver disease, elevated levels of GGT and MCV perform reasonably well for ruling in chronic excessive alcohol exposure, but are beset by poor sensitivity. GGT and MCV become abnormal after several weeks of excessive alcohol use and take up to 6 weeks and 16 weeks, respectively, to normalize after cessation.[7,8] However, these measures are inadequate for alcohol assessment among patients with existing chronic liver disease, which may itself causes GGT and MCV abnormalities.

CDT is a specific transferrin isoform that increases with excessive daily alcohol exposure (50–80 g alcohol per day) owing to alcohol's interference with glycosylation of transferrin.[9] CDT becomes abnormal after approximately 1 week of continuous excessive drinking and normalizes after 2 weeks of abstinence. It is approved by the US Food and Drug Administration as an alcohol biomarker and has an excellent diagnostic accuracy among general patient populations. However, liver disease may falsely elevate CDT, so its diagnostic accuracy declines considerably in the setting of end-stage liver disease—46% to 73% sensitivity and 70% specificity.[10] Also, obesity and active smoking can confound CDT, and false-positive results have been reported among patients with primary biliary cholangitis.[6,9]

PEth is a potentially useful biomarker for the detection of recent moderate to heavy alcohol use, although it is not widely available for clinical use. PEth is one of a group of abnormal phospholipids produced in red cell membranes when exposed to moderate to heavy quantities of alcohol. It is usually tested in whole blood samples, but can also be tested in dried blood samples. It is detectable within 1 hour of and for up to 1 to 4 weeks after moderate to heavy alcohol exposure.[9,11] Liver disease does not affect blood PEth levels. A PEth cutoff of 20 ng/mL had a 100% sensitivity and 96% specificity for alcohol consumption in the prior 1 week among patients before and after undergoing liver transplantation.[12] However, routine clinical use of PEth testing is on hold until further validation and the availability of less expensive and simpler testing methodologies.

Direct Biomarkers

Direct biomarkers measure ethanol or its metabolites in breath, blood, urine, and/or hair. They are best used to assess for recent and ongoing alcohol use. Law enforcement, employer, and insurance entities also use this category of biomarkers in cases requiring appraisal of alcohol use. Ethanol can be directly tested in the blood. However, it has a very short detection window (12 hours) and is thus only useful for proving acute alcohol ingestion. Blood sample handling and storage may affect the accuracy of measurements, either falsely increasing or decreasing the measured alcohol concentration; this factor is particularly important in establishing whether the proper chain of custody has been maintained for a sample required for legal purposes.

Ethyl glucuronide (EtG) and ethyl sulfate are minor alcohol metabolism products that can be detected within 1 hour and to up to 3 days after alcohol consumption.[8] EtG is formed through the conjugation of ethanol with activated glucuronic acid and ethyl sulfate through conjugation of ethanol with sulfate. They are commercially available and not confounded by existing liver disease.[13] A urinary EtG cutoff of 0.5 mg/L detected recent alcohol use with an 89% sensitivity and 99% specificity in a study conducted among patients with end-stage liver disease awaiting organ transplantation.[14] False-positive result may occur owing to exposure to alcohol-containing mouthwashes and hand sanitizers, and false-negative results may result from *Escherichia coli* hydrolysis of EtG with concomitant urinary tract infections and intentional urinary sample dilution (either by direct addition of water or by ingestions of large volumes of water).[10] Therefore, urine creatinine should be assessed concomitantly with a threshold of greater than 20 mg/dL used as a minimum requirement.[11] Also, concomitant testing of EtS, which is not affected by bacterial degradation, provides corroboration of negative urinary EtG results.

Ethyl glucoronide concentration measurement in hair samples allows for the detection of chronic alcohol use up to 3 to 6 months after heavy consumption. The hair sample required is approximately 200 strands (the thickness of a pencil) cut close to the scalp and at least 6 cm in length. Samples less than 3 cm in length may yield inaccurate results. One centimeter of hair reflects approximately 1 month. Based on internationally adopted cutoffs, less than 7 pg EtG/mg hair verifies alcohol abstinence and greater than 30 pg EtG/mg hair indicates chronic excessive drinking (>60 g of ethanol intake per day). Hair EtG concentrations between 7 and 30 pg ETG/mg hair is regarded as an indicator of regular alcohol consumption.[10] In a study conducted among patients with chronic liver disease, hair EtG identified moderate drinking (28 g ethanol daily) with 90% sensitivity and 88% specificity using the 7 pg/mg cutoff and 81% sensitivity and 93% specificity using the 30 pg/mg cutoff.[15] The study further showed that EtG diagnostic accuracy was slightly better among patient with cirrhosis compared with those without. It is important to keep in mind, however, that EtG concentrations may be decreases by hair treatments such as coloring, perming, and thermal straightening.

In summary, the most useful ways to assess for alcohol use in patients with chronic liver disease are testing for urinary EtG, hair EtG, serum PEth, and BAC (**Table 2**). Urinary EtG and BAC are best for the determination of acute alcohol ingestion. PEth seems to be useful for determining recent moderate alcohol use, although further study is required. Hair EtG is the best objective marker of chronic excessive alcohol use. Essentially all of these tests would meet the legal requirements for alcohol testing in most jurisdictions, assuming that, in individual cases, samples are properly handled, the chain of custody is preserved, and the performing laboratory meets quality controls and forensic certification.

Having determined whether the patient in our case scenario has experienced either acute or recent alcohol consumption or both, and recalling that these results were obtained within the context of a medical examination, how should this information be used to protect the patient and promote public safety? The ethical and legal rules of patient—doctor confidentiality encumber the physician from reporting the acute alcohol ingestion or the return to drinking in violation of the court-ordered alcohol abstinence to law enforcement or the court, respectively. Issues surrounding reporting of patient alcohol-related impairment by physicians will follow consideration of another case scenario where this is relevant.

Table 2
Alcohol biomarkers

Biomarker	Duration of Required Ethanol Exposure	Detection Interval Following After Exposure	Confounders	Sensitivity/Specificity in Advanced Chronic Liver Disease	Interpretation
Mean corpuscular volume	8 wk	8–16 wk	• Chronic liver disease • Macrocytic anemia • Hypothyroidism	—	—
Gamma glutamyl transferase	5 wk	2–6 wk	• Chronic liver disease • Hepatotoxic drugs	—	—
Carbohydrate-deficient transferrin	1–2 wk	2–3 wk	• Advanced chronic liver disease • Congenital-glycosylation disorders • Obesity • Smoking	46%–73%/70%	Chronic excessive alcohol intake; can determine relapse
Phosphatidylethanol	1 h	1–4 wk	—	100%/96%	Recent moderate to heavy alcohol use; can determine relapse
Blood alcohol level	Immediately	—	—	—	Acute alcohol intake; can determine relapse
Urinary ethyl glucuronide	1 h	3–4 d	• Alcohol-containing mouthwash/hand sanitizers • *Escherichia coli* urinary tract infection • Dilute urine	89%/99%	Acute alcohol intake; can determine relapse
Hair ethyl glucuronide	—	3–6 mo[16]	Hair treatments	90%/88% using the 7 pg/mg cutoff[15]	Chronic excessive alcohol intake

Data from Refs.[7,8,10]

ASSESSMENT OF ALCOHOL USE IN CIRRHOSIS WITH COVERT OR OVERT HEPATIC ENCEPHALOPATHY

In general, the elimination of alcohol is increasingly impaired with decreasing liver function.[3,17] This factor may result in some patients with cirrhosis becoming significantly impaired with lower amounts of alcohol than those commonly associated with impairment. This factor may be particularly problematic when the patient has fluctuating HE with overt HE (OHE) or more challenging in the presence of CHE. For example, a 56-year-old man presents for follow-up with a history of alcohol-related cirrhosis. He has stopped all alcohol use; he reports feeling well except for some difficulties with sleeping at night. He continues to work as a taxi driver. When tinkering around the house he sometimes feels a bit clumsy. His wife shares that she has noticed his thinking is a bit slower than usual. On examination, he is oriented to person, place, and time, and does not have asterixis; his neurologic examination is intact. This patient's mild memory and sleep difficulties raise the possibility of HE. HE spans a wide set of findings ranging from subclinical to clinically obvious neuropsychiatric deficits. HE may be classified into CHE or OHE based on the absence or presence of gross neuropsychiatric symptoms. When patients manifest gross neuropsychiatric abnormalities, OHE is diagnosed. When the patient has subclinical neuropsychiatric deficits that are clinically imperceptible but apparent on specialized testing, covert HE (CHE; also known as minimal or subclinical) is present.

Overt Hepatic Encephalopathy

OHE, along with variceal bleeding and ascites, is a defining event in the decompensated stage of cirrhosis. OHE is characterized by gross neuropsychiatric abnormalities. Its two earliest clinical markers are asterixis and temporal disorientation.[18] If OHE is untreated it can deteriorate progressively from a state of mild temporal disorientation to gross confusion, somnolence, and finally coma. Because OHE is a state of gross cognitive impairment and an acute medical illness, clinicians are typically comfortable interdicting patients with OHE from driving, working, or engaging in other higher order activities that require complex cognitive function.

Covert Hepatic Encephalopathy

CHE (also known as minimal or subclinical encephalopathy) refers to neuropsychiatric abnormalities occurring in patients with cirrhosis who do not have clinically overt signs of HE. Patients with CHE seems to be grossly normal—meaning that they have a normal level of consciousness, orientation, and seem to be neurologically intact on physical examination—but are impaired on specialized neuropsychiatric testing. CHE occurs in both the compensated and the decompensated stage of cirrhosis and includes both patients who have never had previous OHE as well as those recovering from an OHE episode who have lingering neuropsychological impairments. CHE is common, affecting 55% to 80%[19–21] of patients with cirrhosis. CHE has a characteristic neuropsychiatric profile marked specifically by impairments in attention, visuospatial perception, psychomotor speed, fine motor control, and global IQ.[22–26] Patients with CHE frequently also have difficulty with short-term memory.[27] Verbal ability is preserved in CHE. Although patients with cirrhosis commonly report sleep disturbance, insomnia, and daytime sleepiness, it is not yet clear that these are truly a function of CHE.[28]

CHE has clear implications for public safety. CHE is associated with the risk of impaired driving, a function that requires coordination between several cognitive domains that are impaired in CHE, including reaction time, psychomotor function, and attention. Gitlin and colleagues[29] were among the first to raise concern about the ability of patients with CHE to safely operate heavy machinery based their observations of neuropsychiatric impairments among 37 patients with cirrhosis, 8% of whom had abnormal electroencephalographic findings and 70% of whom had abnormal paper and pencil psychometric testing. Watanabe and colleagues[30] later provided greater support for these concerns when they found that 44% of patients with CHE performed poorly on tests of driving ability. Wein and colleagues[31] evaluated the driving ability of patients with cirrhosis directly using standardized on-road driving tests and found that those with CHE had significantly reduced capacity to drive compared with both subjects with cirrhosis who had no CHE and with noncirrhotic controls. Specifically, patients with CHE had worse performance in several specific driving domains (car handling, adaptation, cautiousness, and maneuvering) and were 10 times more likely to require intervention from the driving instructor to avoid an accident compared with controls. Using a virtual driving simulator among a cohort of patients with cirrhosis, Lauridsen and colleagues[32] identified a greater proportion of unsafe drivers among patients with CHE compared with patients without CHE (16% vs 7%), which persisted at 1 year on follow-up testing (18% vs 0%). An anonymous survey showed that patients with CHE have a greater number of motor vehicle accidents and crashes than patients without.[33] In summary, both simulated and real-life on the road tests have demonstrated that CHE is associated with unfit driving.

Clinicians rarely test for CHE, partly because of the time constraints of a typical office visit and partly because of lack of agreement on the validity or significance of the available tests.[34] Although there are multiple testing strategies, none are routine or have been established as the gold standard clinical test.[35] Furthermore, the tests are often copyrighted, complicated to perform and interpret, and frequently need either specialized training or equipment to conduct. Compounding this is the challenge of identifying who among patients with CHE are unfit to drive and truly at risk for motor vehicle accidents, a task that clinicians are not routinely trained to perform.

Amid this uncertainty, there are 4 CHE tests practical for clinical use: (i) a battery of 4 paper-and-pencil tests consisting of the number connection tests A and B, digit symbol test, and block design test, (ii) the repeatable battery for the assessment of neuropsychological status (RBANS), (iii) the inhibitory control test (ICT) and (iv) the EncephalApp Stroop Test. The 4-test battery is endorsed by expert groups as an alternative to the Psychometric Hepatic Encephalopathy Score, which is the most extensively used CHE test in clinical research studies, but impossible to use in the United States because it is long, copyrighted, and lacks normative reference data for the United States. Abnormalities in 2 of 4 tests (defined as a score 2 of standard deviations below age and education matched controls) is the cutoff for CHE. The 4-test battery is easy to use and incorporates the original psychometric tests that identified CHE-specific neuropsychiatric deficits.[36] However, it may be difficult for clinicians to access and interpret. The RBANS has also been used in studies for CHE diagnosis and is endorsed by the International Society for Hepatic Encephalopathy and Nitrogen Metabolism.[18] Realistically, however, clinicians must refer their patients to a psychologist for RBANS testing because the test is copyrighted, lengthy, and requires specialized training to administer and score. The ICT (www.hecme.tv) is a computerized test of attention and response inhibition that requires patients to respond to the computer screen appearance of specific targets (an X followed by a Y or vice versa), but to inhibit this response upon the appearance of lures (pairs of XX or YYs). Five responses to lures is the cutoff for CHE.[33] The ICT is widely available and easy to use. Its greatest advantage is that it was found to be superior to psychometric testing specifically for predicting motor vehicle crashes in a study conducted among patients with cirrhosis. However, there are concerns that the ICT has insufficient diagnostic accuracy for CHE diagnosis and requires more validation. Finally, the most recently developed and very convenient option is the EncephalApp (www.encephalapp.com), a smartphone application of the Stroop task, a widely used psychological test that evaluates psychomotor speed, attention, and cognitive flexibility. The test requires patients to identify the color of the word, rather than the word itself, that appears on the screen. It is widely available, easy to use, and correlates well with the Psychometric Hepatic Encephalopathy Score testing for CHE. Although more study is required to firmly establish this app's validity for CHE diagnosis, it is an appealing and acceptable option.[35] In summary, the EncephalApp, ICT, and 4-test battery are the most practical in-clinic testing options, with consideration of referral of patients who have abnormal testing for formal RBANS evaluation by a psychologist.

Even after CHE is identified in a patient, it is important to keep in mind that some, although not all, patients are unfit drivers. Consequently, patients deemed to have CHE, by any method, still require further evaluation to determine their fitness to drive. Convincing patients with CHE that a driving evaluation is necessary is often difficult; driving is an important aspect of function and autonomy in our society. Patients tend to be optimistic about their ability to drive, and they often resist formal driving evaluation and compliance with recommendations to stop driving.[37] Given the difficulties of diagnosing CHE and the added difficulties of identifying who among CHE are unfit to drive (or perform other tasks), what are the ethical and legal obligations for the physician to report or warn of the impairment?

REPORTING BY PHYSICIANS OF ALCOHOL-RELATED IMPAIRMENT: THE CONFLICT BETWEEN DUTY TO WARN OR REPORT AND PATIENT CONFIDENTIALITY

Alcohol-related impairments could be regarded as the prototypical example of an issue placing physicians in conflicting ethical and legal roles of patient advocacy and confidentiality versus promoting public safety. Many physicians are not aware that statutory and case law in this area is often vague and not clear, particularly where the reporting of impairment is voluntary.[38] Many countries have established processes for the reporting of disabilities relevant to driver licensing and other activities. However, these often conditions only include disorders or disabilities specified in other rules, such as departments of public safety rules, without provision to cover disorders not specifically enumerated.[38–40] The reporting itself is usually voluntary and indicates the physician may (not must) inform. Even in cases where there is a provision to exempt reporting from the patient physician privilege requirements, case law remains vague and certainly does not prevent the physician from being sued. At least 7 states in the United States (California, Utah, Delaware, Nevada, New Jersey, Oregon, Pennsylvania) require mandatory reporting of impaired drivers for specific disorders, usually focusing on epilepsy, dementia, or other cognitive disorders, but that could include drug or substance abuse or any clinically significant cognitive impairment.[38] In these mandatory reporting states, it is presumed that the physician's protection from liability is very strong because the statutes include sections providing that no civil or criminal action may be brought against any person reporting an impaired driver under the applicable law (see, for example, Section 1518(b) of the Pennsylvania Vehicle Code). However, it is noted that, in Canada, where there has been a move toward mandatory requirements to report unfit drivers, there is variation between the provincial courts as to how the laws should be interpreted and physician's risk of liability may not be absolute.[41]

Generally, doctors are advised that they must assess the situation on a case-by-case basis, balancing public safety against the risk of breaching patient confidentiality. The risk of a motor vehicle accident in a patient with a BAC of 0.09% is increased approximately 1.5 times normal.[3] Does this justify the ethical and legal breach of patient confidentiality? Guidelines like this, promulgated by several medical societies, at first glance do not seem to be helpful, but serve as a starting point for analysis by the physician. In this setting of unclear liability, some recommendations can be made based on general medical ethical and legal principles.

Physicians have an ethical duty to educate and warn patients about harm that may arise from a medical condition or the interventions used to treat it. Accordingly, the most important thing a physician can do for patients with alcohol-related impairment is to educate them about the nature of the problem and obtain their agreement to follow suggestions to stop alcohol, voluntarily refrain from driving or performing other acts, and remain compliant with any alcohol rehabilitation initiatives. These interventions of course also promote public safety because what's good for the goose (the patient) is usually good for the gander (the public). For patients who have a limited understanding of the risks involved with continued alcohol or who are noncompliant, enlisting family support may be undertaken, subject to the limits of patient confidentiality. Documentation of good faith efforts to educate and warn may be very useful as a defense should a third party be harmed as a result of impairment.

If a patient remains resistant to physician suggestions (eg, the patient insists on driving home despite being intoxicated or continues to drive a taxi despite impairment related to CHE), the physician arguably has an ethical responsibility to report the impairment. If the risk of harm to a third party is significant and seems to outweigh substantive privacy concerns, a breach in confidentiality may be justified.[38] A legal case often quoted in this context and used to guide physicians regarding when patient confidentiality may be breached for the sake of public safety, is that of Tarasoff.[42] However, it should be noted that this case involved a psychiatrist learning of a patient's intent to kill his girlfriend. The doctor did not breach confidentiality and the girlfriend was murdered. This case is not likely applicable in settings where the risk of intent and harm may be much less clear and severe. A concern for physicians should be overestimating the risk of harm and underestimating the burden to the patient caused by reporting certain impairments. Anxiety is heightened by the occurrence of litigation, fortunately not common (or at least not commonly reported in legal databases), alleging liability of the physician for failing to warn either the patient or a third party about a patient's alcohol-related impairment.[43]

Although all of this may be as vague as the applicable ethical guidelines and relevant laws, in addition to the recommendations outlined herein, physicians should become familiar with the administrative processes and laws regarding reporting of alcohol-related impairment (in particular regarding fitness to drive and the performance of certain occupations) for the jurisdiction in which they practice. The majority of jurisdictions have voluntary reporting with established processes outlined and usually involving a medical advisory board of some type.[38,44,45] Explicit documentation of all good faith efforts to educate patients and family and promote rehabilitation will not totally eliminate the risk of litigation, but will serve as a strong defense.

REFERENCES

1. Greenfeld LA, Henneberg MA. Victim and offender self-reports of alcohol involvement in crime. Available at: https://pubs.niaaa.nih.gov/publications/arh25-1/20-31.htm. Accessed July 7, 2018.

2. National Institute on Alcohol Abuse and Alcoholism. What is a standard drink? Department of Health and Human Services, National Institutes of Health, National Institute on Alcohol Abuse and Alcoholism; 2016. Available at: https://www.niaaa.nih.gov/alcohol-health/overview-alcohol-consumption/what-standard-drink. Accessed July 7, 2018.

3. Perry PJ, Doroudgar S, Van Dyke P. Ethanol forensic toxicology. J Am Acad Psychiatry Law 2017;45(4):429–38.

4. Vonghia L, Michielsen P, Dom G, et al. Diagnostic challenges in alcohol use disorder and alcoholic liver disease. World J Gastroenterol 2014;20(25):8024–32.

5. Higgins-Biddle JC, Babor TF. A review of the Alcohol Use Disorders Identification Test (AUDIT), AUDIT-C, and USAUDIT for screening in the United States: past issues and future directions. Am J Drug Alcohol Abuse 2018;44(6):578–86.

6. Moyer VA. Screening and behavioral counseling interventions in primary care to reduce alcohol misuse: U.S. preventive services task force recommendation statement. Ann Intern Med 2013;159(3):210–8.

7. Peterson K. Biomarkers for alcohol use and abuse–a summary. Alcohol Res Health 2004;28(1):30–7.

8. Ingall GB. Alcohol biomarkers. Clin Lab Med 2012;32(3):391–406.

9. Nanau RM, Neuman MG. Biomolecules and biomarkers used in diagnosis of alcohol drinking and in monitoring therapeutic interventions. Biomolecules 2015;5(3):1339–85.

10. Allen JP, Wurst FM, Thon N, et al. Assessing the drinking status of liver transplant patients with alcoholic liver disease. Liver Transpl 2013;19(4):369–76.

11. Andresen-Streichert H, Muller A, Glahn A, et al. Alcohol biomarkers in clinical and forensic contexts. Dtsch Arztebl Int 2018;115(18):309–15.

12. Andresen-Streichert H, Beres Y, Weinmann W, et al. Improved detection of alcohol consumption using the novel marker phosphatidylethanol in the transplant setting: results of a prospective study. Transpl Int 2017;30(6):611–20.

13. Singal AK, Bataller R, Ahn J, et al. ACG clinical guideline: alcoholic liver disease. Am J Gastroenterol 2018;113(2):175–94.

14. Staufer K, Andresen H, Vettorazzi E, et al. Urinary ethyl glucuronide as a novel screening tool in patients pre- and post-liver transplantation improves detection of alcohol consumption. Hepatology 2011;54(5):1640–9.

15. Stewart SH, Koch DG, Willner IR, et al. Hair ethyl glucuronide is highly sensitive and specific for detecting moderate-to-heavy drinking in patients with liver disease. Alcohol Alcohol 2013;48(1):83–7.

16. Crunelle CL, Yegles M, Nuijs A, et al. Hair ethyl glucuronide levels as a marker for alcohol use and abuse: a review of the current state of the art. Drug Alcohol Depend 2014;134:1–11.

17. Cederbaum AI. Alcohol metabolism. Clin Liver Dis 2012;16:667–85.

18. Randolph C, Hilsabeck R, Kato A, et al. Neuropsychological assessment of hepatic encephalopathy: ISHEN practice guidelines. Liver Int 2009;29(5):629–35.

19. Maldonado-Garza HJ, Vazquez-Elizondo G, Gaytan-Torres JO, et al. Prevalence of minimal hepatic encephalopathy in cirrhotic patients. Ann Hepatol 2011; 10(Suppl 2):S40–4.

20. Das A, Dhiman RK, Saraswat VA, et al. Prevalence and natural history of subclinical hepatic encephalopathy in cirrhosis. J Gastroenterol Hepatol 2001;16(5):531–5.

21. Ridola L, Cardinale V, Riggio O. The burden of minimal hepatic encephalopathy: from diagnosis to therapeutic strategies. Ann Gastroenterol 2018;31(2):151–64.

22. Weissenborn K. PHES: one label, different goods?! J Hepatol 2008;49(3):308–12.

23. Stewart CA, Enders FT, Schneider N, et al. Development of a three-factor neuro-psychological approach for detecting minimal hepatic encephalopathy. Liver Int 2010;30(6):841–9.
24. Weissenborn K, Ennen JC, Schomerus H, et al. Neuropsychological characterization of hepatic encephalopathy. J Hepatol 2001;34(5):768–73.
25. Weissenborn K, Giewekemeyer K, Heidenreich S, et al. Attention, memory, and cognitive function in hepatic encephalopathy. Metab Brain Dis 2005;20(4):359–67.
26. Amodio P, Montagnese S, Gatta A, et al. Characteristics of minimal hepatic encephalopathy. Metab Brain Dis 2004;19(3–4):253–67.
27. Weissenborn K, Heidenreich S, Giewekemeyer K, et al. Memory function in early hepatic encephalopathy. J Hepatol 2003;39(3):320–5.
28. Montagnese S, Turco M, Amodio P. Hepatic encephalopathy and sleepiness: an interesting connection? J Clin Exp Hepatol 2015;5(Suppl 1):S49–53.
29. Gitlin N, Lewis DC, Hinkley L. The diagnosis and prevalence of subclinical hepatic encephalopathy in apparently healthy, ambulant, non-shunted patients with cirrhosis. J Hepatol 1986;3(1):75–82.
30. Watanabe A, Tuchida T, Yata Y, et al. Evaluation of neuropsychological function in patients with liver cirrhosis with special reference to their driving ability. Metab Brain Dis 1995;10(3):239–48.
31. Wein C, Koch H, Popp B, et al. Minimal hepatic encephalopathy impairs fitness to drive. Hepatology 2004;39(3):739–45.
32. Lauridsen MM, Thacker LR, White MB, et al. In patients with cirrhosis, driving simulator performance is associated with real-life driving. Clin Gastroenterol Hepatol 2016;14(5):747–52.
33. Bajaj JS, Hafeezullah M, Hoffmann RG, et al. Minimal hepatic encephalopathy: a vehicle for accidents and traffic violations. Am J Gastroenterol 2007;102(9):1903–9.
34. Bajaj JS, Etemadian A, Hafeezullah M, et al. Testing for minimal hepatic encephalopathy in the United States: an AASLD survey. Hepatology 2007;45(3):833–4.
35. Vilstrup H, Amodio P, Bajaj J, et al. Hepatic encephalopathy in chronic liver disease: 2014 practice guideline by the American Association for the Study of Liver Diseases and the European Association for the Study of the Liver. Hepatology 2014;60(2):715–35.
36. Amodio P, Bemeur C, Butterworth R, et al. The nutritional management of hepatic encephalopathy in patients with cirrhosis: International Society for Hepatic Encephalopathy and Nitrogen Metabolism Consensus. Hepatology 2013;58(1):325–36.
37. Bajaj JS, Saeian K, Hafeezullah M, et al. Patients with minimal hepatic encephalopathy have poor insight into their driving skills. Clin Gastroenterol Hepatol 2008;6(10):1135–9 [quiz: 1065].
38. Berger JT, Rosner F, Kark P, et al. Reporting by physicians of impaired drivers and potentially impaired drivers. The committee on bioethical issues of the medical society of the state of New York. J Gen Intern Med 2000;15(9):667–72.
39. Tex. Health & safety code § 12.096 (2001).
40. Tex. Health & safety code § 12.098 (1995).
41. Coopersmith HG, Korner-Bitensky NA, Mayo NE. Determining medical fitness to drive: physicians' responsibilities in Canada. CMAJ 1989;140(4):375–8.
42. Tarasoff V. Regents of the University of California, 55 P2d 334 (Cal 1976).

43. Cohen SM, Kim A, Metropulos M. Ahn J. Legal ramifications for physicians of patients who drive with hepatic encephalopathy. Clin Gastroenterol Hepatol 2011; 9(2):156–60.
44. Texas Department of Public Safety. Available at: https://www.dps.texas.gov/DriverLicense/MedicalRevocation.htm. Accessed July 7, 2018.
45. Guide for determining driver limitation. Texas Department of Public Safety. Available at: https://www.txacp.org/files/Guide%20for%20Determining.pdf. Accessed July 7, 2018.

Epidemiology of Alcohol Consumption and Societal Burden of Alcoholism and Alcoholic Liver Disease

Page D. Axley, MD[a], Crit Taylor Richardson, MD[b],
Ashwani K. Singal, MD, MS[c],*

KEYWORDS

- Alcoholic cirrhosis • Alcoholic hepatitis • Liver cirrhosis • Prevalence of disease
- Burden of disease • Epidemiology

KEY POINTS

- Alcohol consumption is a significant cause of mortality, morbidity, and social problems, accounting for approximately 5% of deaths worldwide.
- The World Health Organization's 2010 goal was at least a 10% reduction in the harmful use of alcohol. Instead, the burden of alcohol consumption has continued to increase.
- Abstinence remains the cornerstone of treatment, with an additional need for public awareness on the toxic effects of alcohol use and the implementation of policies to restrict availability of alcohol.
- There is an unmet need for the development of more effective treatment options for patients with alcoholic liver disease.

INTRODUCTION

Alcohol consumption is the third most important preventable cause of any disease after smoking and hypertension.[1] About 38% of adults worldwide and 60% to 70% in the United States report alcohol consumption within the past 12 months.[2] According to the World Health Organization (WHO), alcohol consumption is linked to more than 200 diseases and injury-related health conditions.[2] Alcohol consumption accounts for

Disclosure Statement: There are no conflicts of interest. This work was supported by a faculty development grant from the American College of Gastroenterology to A.K. Singal.
[a] Department of Medicine, University of Alabama at Birmingham, 1720 2nd Avenue South, BDB 327, Birmingham, AL 35294, USA; [b] Division of Gastroenterology and Hepatology, University of Alabama at Birmingham, 1720 2nd Avenue South, BDB 380, Birmingham, AL 35294, USA; [c] Division of Gastroenterology and Hepatology, Porphyria Center, University of Alabama at Birmingham, 1720 2nd Avenue South, BDB 380, Birmingham, AL 35294, USA
* Corresponding author.
E-mail address: ashwanisingal.com@gmail.com

4.2% of the global burden of disease measured in disability-adjusted life years (DALYs), especially among individuals in their most productive years, between the ages of 15 and 59 years.[3] DALYs attributed to alcohol consumption have increased by more than 25% among men and women since 1990.[3]

To understand the impact of alcohol consumption, it is important to have an accurate estimation of alcohol exposure and the burden of alcohol-related disease.[4] In the United States, 1 drink contains 14 g of alcohol. This amount is contained in 12 ounces of beer (5% weight/volume), 5 ounces of wine (8%–10% weight/volume), or 1.5 ounces of hard liquor (40%–45% weight/volume).[5] Approximately 1 in 12 adults report heavy alcohol consumption, defined as consumption of greater than 3 drinks per day in men and greater than 2 drinks per day in women, or engagement in binge drinking (>5 drinks in men and >4 drinks in women over 2 hours).[6] Chronic heavy use of alcohol can lead to hepatic steatosis, alcoholic hepatitis, alcoholic cirrhosis, and liver cancer.[7] Whereas hepatic steatosis and, possibly, fibrosis are potentially reversible on cessation of alcohol use, alcoholic cirrhosis can progress to decompensation and liver cancer despite abstinence.[8] Of the various factors responsible for liver disease, duration and amount of alcohol consumed are the most important factors.[9] Mortality rates from alcoholic cirrhosis closely parallel alcohol consumption prevalence rates worldwide.[10] With the growing burden of alcohol-related disease, there is increased need to develop and implement population-based approaches to reduce the health and social burdens caused by alcohol consumption.

WORLD-WIDE DISTRIBUTION AND HOT SPOTS OF ALCOHOL CONSUMPTION

For epidemiologic purposes, alcohol consumption is traditionally reported per capita, or the amount of alcohol consumed in liters per person.[11] Several limitations in the reporting of per capita alcohol consumption contribute to inaccurate estimates of alcohol use. For example, data on alcohol exposure are often derived from surveys of self-reported consumption that might underestimate true alcohol use.[12] Further, global studies of disease burden frequently use *International Statistical Classification of Diseases and Related Health Problems* (ICD) codes, which are inconsistently used across the world. Use of ICD codes may fail to capture those who do not seek medical care and thus miss a large proportion of these individuals.[13,14] Another limitation relates to the reporting of national consumption figures that rely on calculations of legal sales of alcohol and do not account for illegally produced alcohol.[15] It is estimated that approximately a quarter of the total alcohol consumed globally is unrecorded (**Fig. 1**).[16]

According to the most recent WHO data, average alcohol consumption per person among individuals aged 15 years and older is about 6.2 L of pure alcohol per year or 13.5 g of pure alcohol per day. Given that only 38% of the world's population consumes alcohol, drinkers consume an average of 17 L of pure alcohol annually.[2] In 2015, the global estimated prevalence of heavy episodic alcohol use over the past 30 days was 18.3% among adults.[17]

The highest rates of alcohol consumption are in Eastern Europe and the former Soviet Union at greater than 10 L per capita. In contrast, the lowest drinking rates are reported from the Middle East and Southeast Asia at less than 2.5 L per capita, likely due to significant Islamic populations in these regions of the world (**Fig. 2**). The type of alcohol consumed also varies by geographic region. Globally, the most frequent alcohol consumed is spirits (50.1%), followed by beer (34.8%) and wine (8%).[2]

There are differences in trends of per capita alcohol consumption over time across the world (**Fig. 3**). For example, alcohol consumption in North America remains high

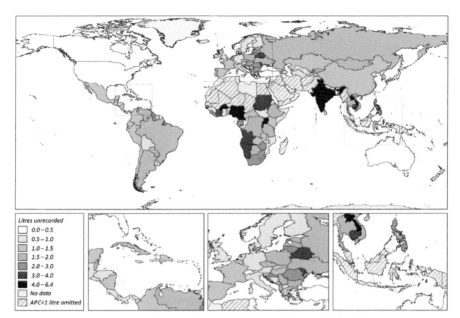

Fig. 1. Proportion of unrecorded alcohol consumption of the total alcohol consumption per capita (APC) in 2015. Countries with less than 1 L of recorded APC were omitted. (*From* Probst C, Manthey J, Merey A, et al. Unrecorded alcohol use: a global modelling study based on nominal group assessments and survey data. Addiction 2018;113(7):1231–41; with permission.)

but has been relatively stable over time.[18] Between 2000 and 2015, among persons older than 18 years of age, alcohol consumption increased by 3% (from 67% to 70%). This was associated with approximately 1% decrease in the prevalence of

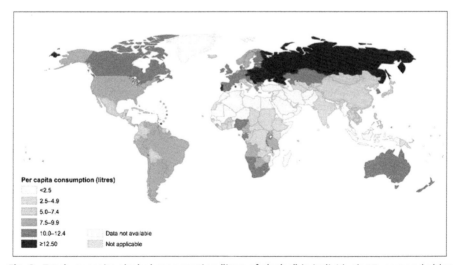

Fig. 2. Total per capita alcohol consumption (liters of alcohol) in individuals 15 years and older in 2010 in WHO member states. (*From* World Health Organization. Global status report on alcohol and health. Geneva (Switzerland): World Health Organization; 2014; with permission.)

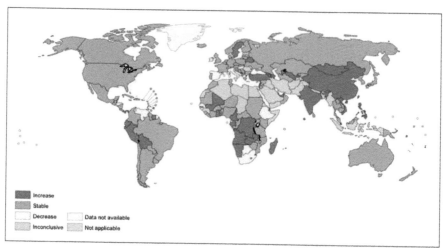

Fig. 3. Five-year change in recorded alcohol per capita among persons aged 15 years and older, 2006 to 2010. (*From* World Health Organization. Global status report on alcohol and health. Geneva (Switzerland): World Health Organization; 2014; with permission.)

alcohol use disorder in this population (from 7.4% to 6.2%).[18,19] Similarly, data from National Institute on Alcohol Abuse and Alcoholism demonstrated a decrease in alcohol consumption from the 1980s to mid-1990s, followed by a slight uptrend from 8.1 L per year in 1990 to 8.9 L per year in 2016.[20] Although consumption has remained relatively stable in the United States, binge drinking has significantly increased, particularly among women.[21]

On the other hand, many Asian countries, such as India and China, are experiencing a significant increase in per capita alcohol consumption, with more than 90% of their alcohol consumption in the form of spirits.[22] Per capita alcohol use by adults in India increased by 107% from 1970 to 1996.[23] This trend has continued into the twenty-first century with the per capita alcohol consumption increasing from 3.6 L to 4.4 L in 2010,[2] and a growing culture of heavy and binge drinking among younger adults.[24] Similarly, in China, per capita alcohol consumption increased from 4.9 L to 6.7 L between 2003 and 2010, with about 70% in the form of spirits.[2] Because greater than 50% of alcohol consumption per capita is unrecorded in Southeast Asia, these figures likely underestimate true alcohol consumption.[22] The trend in increased alcohol consumption in these countries is expected to continue on the background of increased disposable incomes, limited alcohol control policies, and aggressive alcohol marketing strategies.[2,25] Furthermore, demographic patterns in alcohol consumption are also expected to continue, with increased use among younger people and women.[26]

SOCIETAL COST OF ALCOHOLIC LIVER DISEASE

The burden of alcohol use and alcohol use disorders contributes significantly to the health care costs for alcohol-related diseases. For example, patients with alcoholic liver disease (ALD) incur direct costs to the health care system for medical care, and indirect costs to society due to a loss of workforce productivity, absenteeism, injury, early retirement, and mortality.[27] Costs related to alcohol consumption have been estimated at 125 billion Euros in the European Union in 2003[28] and 249 billion dollars in the United States in 2010[29] (these figures account for 1.3%–3.3% of gross domestic product, respectively).[27,30] With an estimated 223.5 billion dollars spent on alcohol abuse in 2006, the societal cost is estimated at $1.90 per individual alcoholic beverage consumed.[31]

Data from the Centers for Disease Control in the United States attributed an average annual number of 87,798 deaths to alcohol between 2006 and 2010, which accounts for 1 in 10 deaths among adults aged 18 to 65 years. This was associated with 2,560,290 years of potential life lost.[32] Age standardized death rates due to alcohol in the United States increased by 17.5% between 1990 and 2016, with 2.89 deaths per 100,000 persons in 2016.[33] Alcohol consumption has also had a significantly global impact on mortality. For example, 3.3 million deaths, or 5.9% of all deaths worldwide, were attributable to alcohol consumption in 2012.[2]

A large portion of the disease burden associated with alcohol use and mortality is due to ALD. For example, the US mortality rate from any cirrhosis increased by 8.2% between 2000 and 2013, from 9.7 to 10.5 deaths per 100,000. Based on the cause of the cirrhosis, the mortality increase over time was much higher for alcohol-related cirrhosis, with an 18.6% increase from 4.3 to 5.1 deaths per 100,000 people.[34] ALD contributed to 48% of all hospitalizations and cirrhosis-related deaths in the United States,[35] with 76% of these affecting individuals aged 25 to 34 years.[34] Transplantation for ALD is also increasing[36] and has now surpassed hepatitis C virus infection as the most common indication for liver transplantation in the United States.[37]

Alcoholic hepatitis, a unique presentation among individuals with chronic active heavy alcohol consumption, presents with acute-on-chronic liver failure and contributes significantly to the morbidity, health care burden, and mortality from ALD.[38,39] Analysis of the National Inpatient Sample database showed that average length of stay and hospital charges in 2010 per hospital admission for alcoholic hepatitis were 6.1 days and $46,264, respectively.[40] In another study on a cohort of 15,496 subjects hospitalized for alcoholic hepatitis, about $2 billion was spent in the 5-year follow-up from 2006 to 2010.[41]

The burden of ALD in Europe is considerably higher than in the United States and is estimated to be the highest in the world.[42,43] In the European Union, one-fifth of the population older than the age of 15 years reports binge drinking (5 or more drinks on an occasion) at least once a week.[44] Currently, it is estimated that 70% of the adults in the WHO European region drink alcohol, consuming an average of 10.7 L annually.[45] An analysis of mortality data from 14 European Union countries demonstrated that a 1 L increase in per capita consumption was associated with a 10% increase in cirrhosis diagnoses.[46]

In the United Kingdom, liver disease is the third leading cause of death before age 75 years, and alcohol contributes to 75% of liver disease mortality.[47] A recent report from the Lancet Standing Commission on liver disease in the United Kingdom projected that ALD will shortly overtake ischemic heart disease with regard to years of working life lost (before the age of 65 years).[48] The National Health Service spends approximately £21 billion annually related to alcohol misuse,[48] and £3.5 billion annually on complications related to ALD.[49] In 2015, there were 1.1 million alcohol-related hospital admissions, representing 7% of total hospital admissions.[48] Admissions for ALD to intensive care units tripled in the United Kingdom over the 10 years from 1996 to 2005.[50] In Portugal, 84% of hospital admissions for cirrhosis to all state hospitals from 1993 to 2008 were related to ALD, with a disproportionate increase in admissions for cirrhosis in men aged 40 to 54 years. Patients with ALD had longer length of stay and increased mortality.[51] Across Europe, prevalence and mortality data indicate that increasing rates of cirrhosis in Europe are linked to dramatic increases in harmful alcohol consumption, most notably in Northern European countries.[52]

China shares the worldwide burden of liver disease with an estimated 300 million people suffering from liver disease.[53] Although chronic viral hepatitis remains the largest cause of liver disease in China, alcohol use disorders are increasing on the background of increased screening and treatment programs for viral hepatitis.[54] Although nationwide large-scale epidemiologic data for ALD are unavailable, the prevalence as reported from specific regions of China ranges from 2.3% to 6.1% of the total population.[55] In a large tertiary referral hospital in Beijing, patients hospitalized with ALD continuously increased from 1.7% in 2002% to 4.6% in 2013, and hospitalizations for severe alcoholic hepatitis increased 2.43 times over the same period.[56] The annual incidence of hospitalizations related to ALD relative to other types of liver disease is growing steadily and an increased number of patients are undergoing liver transplantation for ALD.[55,57]

Of more than 1 million deaths (2% of all deaths) worldwide from cirrhosis,[58] 493,300 (47.9%) were due to ALD, which contributes to 1.2% of all deaths in men and 0.7% of deaths in women.[59] Proportion of cirrhosis deaths due to alcohol is highest in Central Europe at 72.3% and lowest in the Middle East and Northern Africa at 15.9% and 14%, respectively.[59]

POPULATION APPROACHES TO REDUCE ALCOHOLISM

Regional variations in the incidence and burden of ALD influence population-based strategies to reduce its burden. Taken together, these data underscore the current unmet need for strategies to reduce the disease burden from alcohol consumption. WHO-endorsed research has shown that the most economical public policy interventions to reduce alcohol-related mortality are taxation of alcoholic beverages, restricting the availability of alcoholic beverages, and imposing bans or restrictions on alcohol advertising.[60]

In most countries, the purchase of alcohol is limited by its availability and laws restricting sales to individuals below a certain minimum age.[61] Price is an important determinant of sales and, ultimately, consumption of alcohol.[62] There is strong evidence that affordability and availability of alcohol drive its consumption.[63–65] Examples of this association are demonstrated by areas of Europe with strong relationships in mortality rates from ALD tied to strategies to limit alcohol availability. For example, in Iceland, the deregulation of beer sales in 1989 was associated with a steady increase in rates of consumption and subsequent increase in mortality from ALD.[66] A study of alcohol consumption in Russia highlights a link between socioeconomic events that correlate with the availability and affordability of alcohol and overall mortality.[67] With the fall of the Soviet Union and the removal of state monopoly in 1992, alcohol consumption and alcohol-attributed disease burden increased significantly, contributing to 50% of all-cause mortality.[68] In 2006, policy changes in Russia, including restricting sale locations and regulations on licensing for producers and distributors, has led to a steady reduction in overall harms from excess alcohol consumption, including the risks of liver-related mortality.[69]

The use of taxation and minimum unit pricing to increase the cost of alcohol are effective approaches to curb excess alcohol consumption.[70,71] For example, in Taiwan the alcohol retail price increased by 7-fold after implementing significant increase in taxation of alcohol-related products in 2002. This resulted in an immediate decrease in alcoholic consumption and a significant reduction in hospital inpatient charges for alcohol-attributable diseases.[72] Regions in Canada have also implemented policies to increase the cost of alcohol, with an appreciable effect on alcohol-related mortality. In British Columbia, between 2002 and 2009, alcohol-related mortality decreased by 32% after the implementation of a 10% increase in the minimum unit price of all alcoholic beverages.[73] Minimum unit pricing has recently been passed into law in Scotland after ongoing legal challenges by the alcohol industry.[74] It is estimated that with a 50 pence minimum alcohol consumption will decrease by 3.5%, leading to 120 fewer alcohol attributable deaths, 1200 fewer hospital admissions, and a saving of £12.1 million each year.[75]

There are several other population-based approaches for limiting alcohol consumption, including use of a legal drinking age,[76] regulation in the number of alcohol selling outlets,[77] and restricting alcohol sales to certain hours of the day or days of the week.[78] Governments have also employed monopolies with licensing power to control the supply and availability of alcoholic beverages.[79] Laws against drinking and driving and public intoxication have also been implemented to curb the consumption of alcohol.[80] In many countries, advertisements on alcohol have been shown to drive increase in alcohol consumption, with an unhealthy pattern of drinking.[81,82] Exposure to alcohol marketing is associated with earlier drinking age, increased initiation of drinking, and heightened drinking intensity among current drinkers.[83,84] Data from the WHO in 2012 from 159 countries showed that nearly 40% of countries had no restrictions on alcohol marketing policies in place, with little change from 2002 to 2012.[2,85] On the other end of the spectrum, approximately 10% of countries located in the predominantly Islamic regions of northern Africa and the Middle East, reported a complete ban to reduce exposure to alcohol marketing.[2] Alcohol marketing restrictions have been successful in minimizing the allure of alcohol, particularly in vulnerable populations.[86] However, the most cost-effective policies and interventions to reduce alcohol consumption are limiting alcohol sale availability or increasing alcohol price.[87]

SUMMARY

Trends in the epidemiology of ALD reflect the current burden of disease and underscore the need for effective strategies to combat harmful alcohol use and management of ALD. The best current therapy remains complete abstinence of alcohol.[88–91] Alcohol consumption and the incidence of ALD are expected to continue to increase in the upcoming decades on the background of limited effective pharmacologic therapies for this disease.[92] Clearly, there remains an unmet need for the development of other effective treatment options for patients with ALD. With increased research efforts, there may be new treatment options, as well as strategies, to reduce alcohol consumption. Population-based approaches can affect the consumption of alcohol with direct health benefits and cost savings. Advances in medical therapies and worldwide reduction of harmful alcohol use are desperately needed to curtail the growing global burden of ALD and to achieve the WHO target of 3 to 4 alcohol-related deaths per 100,000 people.[1]

REFERENCES

1. Singal AK, Anand BS. Epidemiology of ALD. Clin Liv Dis 2013;2(2):53–6.
2. World Health Organization. Global status report on alcohol and health. Geneva (Switzerland): World Health Organization; 2014.
3. Gakidou E, Afshin A, Abajobir AA, et al. Global, regional, and national comparative risk assessment of 84 behavioural, environmental and occupational, and metabolic risks or clusters of risks, 1990–2016: a systematic analysis for the Global Burden of Disease Study 2016. Lancet 2017;390(10100):1345–422.
4. Immunological abnormalities in ALD. Lancet 1983;2(8350):605–6.

5. Mandayam S, Jamal MM, Morgan TR. Epidemiology of ALD. Semin Liver Dis 2004;24(3):217–32.

6. Rehm J, Gmel GE Sr, Gmel G, et al. The relationship between different dimensions of alcohol use and the burden of disease-an update. Addiction 2017; 112(6):968–1001.

7. Crawford JM. Histologic findings in ALD. Clin Liver Dis 2012;16(4):699–716.

8. Bataller R, Gao B. Liver fibrosis in ALD. Semin Liver Dis 2015;35(2):146–56.

9. Becker U, Deis A, Sorensen TI, et al. Prediction of risk of liver disease by alcohol intake, sex, and age: a prospective population study. Hepatology 1996;23(5): 1025–9.

10. Stein E, Cruz-Lemini M, Altamirano J, et al. Heavy daily alcohol intake at the population level predicts the weight of alcohol in cirrhosis burden worldwide. J Hepatol 2016;65(5):998–1005.

11. Bloomfield K, Stockwell T, Gmel G, et al. International comparisons of alcohol consumption. Alcohol Res Health 2003;27(1):95–109.

12. Ramstedt M. How much alcohol do you buy? A comparison of self-reported alcohol purchases with actual sales. Addiction 2010;105(4):649–54.

13. World Health Organization. Alcohol and Injuries. Emergency department studies in an international perspective. In: Cherpitel CJ, Borges G, Hungerford D, et al, editors. Room R. The relation between blood alcohol content and clinically assessed intoxication: lessons from applying the ICD-10 Y90 and Y91 codes in the emergency room. France: WHO; 2009. p. 135–46.

14. Faiad Y, Khoury B, Daouk S, et al. Frequency of use of the *International Classification of Diseases* ICD-10 diagnostic categories for mental and behavioural disorders across world regions. Epidemiol Psychiatr Sci 2017;1–9. https://doi.org/ 10.1017/S2045796017000683.

15. Greenfield TK, Kerr WC. Tracking alcohol consumption over time. Alcohol Res Health 2003;27(1):30–8.

16. Probst C, Manthey J, Merey A, et al. Unrecorded alcohol use: a global modelling study based on nominal group assessments and survey data. Addiction 2018; 113(7):1231–41.

17. Peacock A, Leung J, Larney S, et al. Global statistics on alcohol, tobacco and illicit drug use: 2017 status report. Addiction 2018;113(10):1905–26.

18. Kim W. Burden of liver disease in the United States: summary of a workshop. Hepatology 2002;36(1):227–42.

19. Liver transplantation for alcoholic liver disease. Proceedings of a meeting. Bethesda, Maryland, December 6-7, 1996. Liver Transpl Surg 1997;3(3):197–350.

20. Role of iron in alcoholic liver disease. Proceedings of a symposium. October, 2002. Bethesda, Maryland, USA. Alcohol 2003;30(2):91–158.

21. Dwyer-Lindgren L, Flaxman AD, Ng M, et al. Drinking patterns in US counties from 2002 to 2012. Am J Public Health 2015;105(6):1120–7.

22. Proceedings of the international symposium on alcoholic liver and pancreatic diseases and cirrhosis, 18-19 May 2006, Marina del Rey, California, USA. J Gastroenterol Hepatol 2006;21(Suppl 3):S1–110.

23. Das SK, Balakrishnan V, Vasudevan DM. Alcohol: its health and social impact in India. Natl Med J India 2006;19(2):94–9.

24. Bhattacharyya M, Barman NN, Goswami B. Survey of alcohol-related cirrhosis at a tertiary care center in North East India. Indian J Gastroenterol 2016;35(3): 167–72.

25. Jiang H, Xiang X, Hao W, et al. Measuring and preventing alcohol use and related harm among young people in Asian countries: a thematic review. Glob Health Res Policy 2018;3:14.
26. Rehm J, Roerecke M. Patterns of drinking and liver cirrhosis – what do we know and where do we go? J Hepatol 2015;62(5):1000–1.
27. Laramée P, Kusel J, Leonard S, et al. The economic burden of alcohol dependence in Europe. Alcohol Alcohol 2013;48(3):259–69.
28. Anderson P, Baumberg B. Alcohol policy: who should sit at the table? Addiction 2007;102(2):335–6.
29. Sacks JJ, Gonzales KR, Bouchery EE, et al. 2010 National and State costs of excessive alcohol consumption. Am J Prev Med 2015;49(5):e73–9.
30. Rehm J, Mathers C, Popova S, et al. Global burden of disease and injury and economic cost attributable to alcohol use and alcohol-use disorders. Lancet 2009;373(9682):2223–33.
31. Bouchery EE, Harwood HJ, Sacks JJ, et al. Economic costs of excessive alcohol consumption in the U.S., 2006. Am J Prev Med 2011;41(5):516–24.
32. Stahre M, Roeber J, Kanny D, et al. Contribution of excessive alcohol consumption to deaths and years of potential life lost in the United States. Prev Chronic Dis 2014;11:E109.
33. Mokdad AH, Ballestros K, Echko M, et al. The state of US health, 1990-2016. JAMA 2018;319(14):1444.
34. Nemtsov AV. Alcohol-related human losses in Russia in the 1980s and 1990s. Addiction 2002;97(11):1413–25.
35. Singal AK, Salameh H, Kamath PS. Prevalence and in-hospital mortality trends of infections among patients with cirrhosis: a nationwide study of hospitalised patients in the United States. Aliment Pharmacol Ther 2014;40(1):105–12.
36. Kling CE, Perkins JD, Carithers RL, et al. Recent trends in liver transplantation for ALD in the United States. World J Hepatol 2017;9(36):1315–21.
37. Cholankeril G, Ahmed A. Alcoholic liver disease replaces hepatitis C virus infection as the leading indication for liver transplantation in the United States. Clin Gastroenterol Hepatol 2018;16:1356.
38. Singal AK, Kamath PS, Gores GJ, et al. Alcoholic hepatitis: current challenges and future directions. Clin Gastroenterol Hepatol 2014;12(4):555–64 [quiz: e31–2].
39. Lucey MR, Mathurin P, Morgan TR. Alcoholic hepatitis. N Engl J Med 2009; 360(26):2758–69.
40. Jinjuvadia R, Liangpunsakul S. Trends in alcoholic hepatitis related hospitalizations, financial burden, and mortality in the United States. J Clin Gastroenterol 2015;49(6):506–11.
41. Thompson JA, Martinson N, Martinson M. Mortality and costs associated with alcoholic hepatitis: a claims analysis of a commercially insured population. Alcohol 2018;71:57–63.
42. Abenavoli L, Milic N, Capasso F. Anti-oxidant therapy in non-alcoholic fatty liver disease: the role of silymarin. Endocrine 2012;42(3):754–5.
43. Abenavoli L, Milic N, De Lorenzo A, et al. A pathogenetic link between non-alcoholic fatty liver disease and celiac disease. Endocrine 2013;43(1):65–7.
44. Bräker AB, Soellner R. Alcohol drinking cultures of European adolescents. Eur J Public Health 2016;26(4):581–6.
45. Abenavoli L, Scarpellini E, Rouabhia S, et al. Probiotics in non-alcoholic fatty liver disease: which and when. Ann Hepatol 2013;12(3):357–63.

46. Ramstedt M. Per capita alcohol consumption and liver cirrhosis mortality in 14 European countries. Addiction 2002;96(1s1):19–33.
47. Williams R, Aspinall R, Bellis M, et al. Addressing liver disease in the UK: a blueprint for attaining excellence in health care and reducing premature mortality from lifestyle issues of excess consumption of alcohol, obesity, and viral hepatitis. Lancet 2014;384(9958):1953–97.
48. Williams R, Alexander G, Armstrong I, et al. Disease burden and costs from excess alcohol consumption, obesity, and viral hepatitis: fourth report of the lancet standing commission on liver disease in the UK. Lancet 2018;391(10125):1097–107.
49. Hazeldine S, Hydes T, Sheron N. ALD - the extent of the problem and what you can do about it. Clin Med 2015;15(2):179–85.
50. Welch C, Harrison D, Short A, et al. The increasing burden of ALD on United Kingdom critical care units: secondary analysis of a high quality clinical database. J Health Serv Res Policy 2008;13(Suppl 2):40–4.
51. Marinho RT, Duarte H, Gíria J, et al. The burden of alcoholism in fifteen years of cirrhosis hospital admissions in Portugal. Liver Int 2014;35(3):746–55.
52. Pimpin L, Cortez-Pinto H, Negro F, et al. Burden of liver disease in Europe: epidemiology and analysis of risk factors to identify prevention policies. J Hepatol 2018;69(3):718–35.
53. Fan JG. Epidemiology of alcoholic and nonalcoholic fatty liver disease in China. J Gastroenterol Hepatol 2013;28(Suppl 1):11–7.
54. Zheng X, Wang J, Yang D. Antiviral therapy for chronic hepatitis B in China. Med Microbiol Immunol 2015;204:115–20.
55. Wang F-S, Fan J-G, Zhang Z, et al. The global burden of liver disease: the major impact of China. Hepatology 2014;60(6):2099–108.
56. Huang A, Chang B, Sun Y, et al. Disease spectrum of ALD in Beijing 302 Hospital from 2002 to 2013: a large tertiary referral hospital experience from 7422 patients. Medicine 2017;96(7):e6163.
57. Wang W, Xu Y, Jiang C, et al. Advances in the treatment of severe alcoholic hepatitis. Curr Med Res Opin 2018;1–29. https://doi.org/10.1080/03007995.2018.
58. Rehm J, Samokhvalov AV, Shield KD. Global burden of ALDs. J Hepatol 2013;59(1):160–8.
59. Lozano R, Naghavi M, Foreman K, et al. Global and regional mortality from 235 causes of death for 20 age groups in 1990 and 2010: a systematic analysis for the Global Burden of Disease Study 2010. Lancet 2012;380(9859):2095–128.
60. Sornpaisarn BSK, Österberg E, Rehm J. Resource tool on alcohol taxation and pricing policies. Geneva (Switzerland): World Health Organization; 2017.
61. Babor TF, Caetano R, Casswell S, et al. Alcohol: no ordinary commodity. Oxford (UK): Oxford University Press; 2010.
62. Gallet CA. The demand for alcohol: a meta-analysis of elasticities. Aust J Agr Resource Econ 2007;51(2):121–35.
63. Sheron N. Alcohol and liver disease in Europe – simple measures have the potential to prevent tens of thousands of premature deaths. J Hepatol 2016;64(4):957–67.
64. Anderson P, Chisholm D, Fuhr DC. Effectiveness and cost-effectiveness of policies and programmes to reduce the harm caused by alcohol. Lancet 2009;373(9682):2234–46.
65. Elder RW, Lawrence B, Ferguson A, et al. The effectiveness of tax policy interventions for reducing excessive alcohol consumption and related harms. Am J Prev Med 2010;38(2):217–29.

66. Tyrfingsson T, Olafsson S, Bjornsson ES, et al. Alcohol consumption and liver cirrhosis mortality after lifting ban on beer sales in country with state alcohol monopoly: table 1. Eur J Public Health 2014;25(4):729–31.

67. Zaridze D, Lewington S, Boroda A, et al. Alcohol and mortality in Russia: prospective observational study of 151 000 adults. Lancet 2014;383(9927):1465–73.

68. Zaridze D, Brennan P, Boreham J, et al. Alcohol and cause-specific mortality in Russia: a retrospective case–control study of 48 557 adult deaths. Lancet 2009;373(9682):2201–14.

69. Neufeld M, Rehm J. Alcohol consumption and mortality in Russia since 2000: are there any changes following the alcohol policy changes starting in 2006? Alcohol Alcohol 2013;48(2):222–30.

70. Jiang H, Room R. Action on minimum unit pricing of alcohol: a broader need. Lancet 2018;391(10126):1157.

71. Meier PS, Holmes J, Angus C, et al. Estimated effects of different alcohol taxation and price policies on health inequalities: a mathematical modelling study. PLoS Med 2016;13(2):e1001963.

72. Lin CM, Liao CM. Inpatient expenditures on alcohol-attributed diseases and alcohol tax policy: a nationwide analysis in Taiwan from 1996 to 2010. Public Health 2014;128(11):977–84.

73. Zhao J, Stockwell T, Martin G, et al. The relationship between minimum alcohol prices, outlet densities and alcohol-attributable deaths in British Columbia, 2002-09. Addiction 2013;108(6):1059–69.

74. Gilmore W, Chikritzhs T, Stockwell T, et al. Alcohol: taking a population perspective. Nat Rev Gastroenterol Hepatol 2016;13(7):426–34.

75. Meier P, Brennan A, Angus C, et al. Minimum unit pricing for alcohol clears final legal hurdle in Scotland. BMJ 2017;359:j5372.

76. Plunk AD, Krauss MJ, Syed-Mohammed H, et al. The impact of the minimum legal drinking age on alcohol-related chronic disease mortality. Alcohol Clin Exp Res 2016;40(8):1761–8.

77. Gmel G, Holmes J, Studer J. Are alcohol outlet densities strongly associated with alcohol-related outcomes? A critical review of recent evidence. Drug Alcohol Rev 2016;35(1):40–54.

78. Holmes J, Guo Y, Maheswaran R, et al. The impact of spatial and temporal availability of alcohol on its consumption and related harms: a critical review in the context of UK licensing policies. Drug Alcohol Rev 2014;33(5):515–25.

79. Hahn RA, Middleton JC, Elder R, et al. Effects of alcohol retail privatization on excessive alcohol consumption and related harms: a community guide systematic review. Am J Prev Med 2012;42(4):418–27.

80. Esser MB, Bao J, Jernigan DH, et al. Evaluation of the evidence base for the alcohol industry's actions to reduce drink driving globally. Am J Public Health 2016;106(4):707–13.

81. Hollingworth W, Ebel BE, McCarty CA, et al. Prevention of deaths from harmful drinking in the United States: the potential effects of tax increases and advertising bans on young drinkers. J Stud Alcohol 2006;67(2):300–8.

82. Esser MB, Jernigan DH. Policy approaches for regulating alcohol marketing in a global context: a public health perspective. Annu Rev Public Health 2018;39(1):385–401.

83. Jernigan D, Noel J, Landon J, et al. Alcohol marketing and youth alcohol consumption: a systematic review of longitudinal studies published since 2008. Addiction 2017;112(Suppl 1):7–20.

84. Chang F-c, Lee C-m, Chen P-h, et al. Using media exposure to predict the initiation and persistence of youth alcohol use in Taiwan. Int J Drug Policy 2014;25(3): 386–92.

85. Esser MB, Jernigan DH. Assessing restrictiveness of national alcohol marketing policies. Alcohol Alcohol 2014;49(5):557–62.

86. Babor TF, Jernigan D, Brookes C, et al. Toward a public health approach to the protection of vulnerable populations from the harmful effects of alcohol marketing. Addiction 2017;112:125–7.

87. Martineau F, Tyner E, Lorenc T, et al. Population-level interventions to reduce alcohol-related harm: an overview of systematic reviews. Prev Med 2013;57(4): 278–96.

88. Guirguis J, Chhatwal J, Dasarathy J, et al. Clinical impact of alcohol-related cirrhosis in the next decade: estimates based on current epidemiological trends in the United States. Alcohol Clin Exp Res 2015;39(11):2085–94.

89. Singal AK, Kodali S, Vucovich LA, et al. Diagnosis and treatment of alcoholic hepatitis: a systematic review. Alcohol Clin Exp Res 2016;40(7):1390–402.

90. Louvet A, Labreuche J, Artru F, et al. Main drivers of outcome differ between short and long-term in severe alcoholic hepatitis: a prospective study. Hepatology 2017;66(5):1464–73.

91. Thursz MR, Forrest EH, Ryder S, et al. Prednisolone or pentoxifylline for alcoholic hepatitis. N Engl J Med 2015;373(3):282–3.

92. Singal AK, Bataller R, Ahn J, et al. ACG clinical guideline: ALD. Am J Gastroenterol 2018;113(2):175–94.

Adolescent Alcoholic Liver Disease

Sharonda Alston Taylor, MD, Tamir Miloh, MD*

KEYWORDS

- Alcoholic liver disease (ALD) • Adolescent • Alcohol use • Alcohol dependence
- ALD is becoming more prevalent in young adults
- Alcohol use in pregnancy may lead to fetal alcohol spectrum disorder

KEY POINTS

- Alcohol use is rising in adolescents and young adults.
- Risk of alcohol dependence increases with genetic and psychosocial problems.
- The CAGE questionnaire may be useful for screening.
- Nonalcoholic fatty liver disease (NAFLD) is the most common chronic liver condition and exacerbated by alcohol use and obesity.

Alcohol use is common during adolescence. Data from the 2015 Centers for Disease Control Youth Risk Behavior Surveillance System survey among middle school students in the United States and its territories showed that 13% to 41.3% ever drank alcohol and 8% to 14.1% of adolescents had onset prior to age 11.[1] By high school, 63.2% of students surveyed drank at least 1 drink (more than a few sips) at least 1 day in their life.[1] In the Monitoring the Future study, the 2017 prevalence rates of alcohol use for eighth, tenth, and twelfth graders were 23.1%, 42.2%, and 61.5%, respectively.[2] Adolescent alcohol use is a global problem that varies by region with the World Health Organization (WHO) European Region, with WHO Region of the Americas having highest overall percent of current adolescent (15–19 years of age) drinkers, although no region lacks alcohol use.[3]

Although many adolescents use alcohol, the risk of alcohol dependence increases based on genetic and psychosocial factors. Genetic factors include parental and familial alcohol use disorders (AUDs), polymorphisms in dopamine receptor genes, and alterations in genes responsible for dopamine and alcohol degradation. These alterations may result in variable levels of intoxication, tolerance, and dependence on

The authors have nothing to disclose.
Department of Pediatrics, Texas Children's Hospital, 6701 Fannin Street, Houston, TX 77030, USA
* Corresponding author.
E-mail address: Tamir.miloh@bcm.edu

alcohol. Psychosocial factors contributing to AUDs include parental role modeling of alcohol use; parental attitudes toward alcohol; parenting styles (especially permissive or authoritarian parenting); accessibility of alcohol; unmet and/or concomitant mental health needs, such as impulsivity, schizophrenia, and bipolar disorder; and age of drinking onset. Onset of AUD peaks during the late teen years to early 20s; however, onset of use prior to 14 years of age can lead to severe medical outcomes and increased risk of alcohol dependence and abuse.[3] Studies suggest that environmental factors may be more significant than genetics in the development of AUDs, but both factors are believed to play a role.[4]

Unique characteristics of adolescent AUDs are (1) the vulnerability of the developing brain to stimulation of the dopaminergic reward system; (2) normative adolescent experimentation and risk-taking behaviors; (3) perception that alcohol consumption is an adult behavior; and (4) increasing influence of peers on decision making. A concerning behavior associated with adolescent AUDs is binge drinking, or heavy episodic drinking (HED), defined as 5 or more drinks consumed in 1 setting; 17.7% of high school–aged drinkers reported HED in past 30 days; worldwide, HED (defined by the WHO as consuming $\geq$60 g of pure alcohol on at least 1 single occasion at least monthly) is much greater among 15 year olds to 19 year olds than in adults.[1,3] Ingestion of large quantities of alcohol at any single time results in increased likelihood of intoxication and in higher dopaminergic response, thus increasing the likelihood of tolerance and dependence. In addition, large quantities of alcohol may cause acute organ damage, notably to the liver and pancreas.

If a provider is concerned about use of alcohol, screening is recommended. Two options for alcohol and drug screening are the CAGE and CRAFFT questionnaires. These can be quickly asked during an office visit and require less time than the HEADDSSS psychosocial screening tool commonly used in pediatric and adolescent medicine.[5] The CAGE questionnaire is a 4-question alcohol-specific screener (**Box 1**). A score of 2 or more on the CAGE questionnaire suggests probable alcoholism.[6] The CRAFFT questionnaire asks 9 questions to screen for alcohol and substance use in the prior 12 months. The higher the score, the higher the risk of a substance use disorder. The CRAFFT self-administered and clinician interview questionnaires are available at www.ceasar.org.

The National Health and Nutrition Examination Survey reported that in adolescents and young adults, nonalcoholic fatty liver disease (NAFLD) is the most common cause of liver disease, accounting for 22% of all chronic liver disease in the later period. The prevalence of alcoholic liver disease (ALD) has been steadily increasing throughout the years: 2.3% between 1988 and 1994, 4.4% between 1999 and 2005, and 5.1% between 2007 and 2012.[7] The British Liver Trust (http://www.britishlivertrust.org.uk/home.aspx) reported that the 2 fastest growing causes of liver damage among

---

Box 1
CAGE questionnaire for alcoholism

1. Have you ever felt the need to *Cut* down on your drinking?

2. Have people *Annoyed* you by criticizing your drinking?

3. Have you ever felt bad or *Guilty* about your drinking?

4. Have you ever had a drink first thing in the morning to steady you nerves or to get rid of a hangover (*Eye opener*)?

Two or more affirmative answers is considered probable alcoholism.

younger people are obesity and alcohol, and the number of young people dying from ALD has increased 8-fold in the past 10 years. NAFLD is present in 2.6% to 9.8% of children and adolescents and in up to 74% among obese individuals. Adolescence is around the legal age for alcohol consumption. NAFLD and metabolic factors are increasingly observed in childhood and adolescence with a trend toward increased exposure to excessive amounts of alcohol, including the binge modality. NAFLD and ALD effects may be synergistic and may hasten progression of liver disease due to the presence of factors predisposing to inflammation and fibrosis.[8] Drinking alcohol during adolescence predisposes to severe liver disease in adulthood. Alcohol consumption was associated with an increased risk of development of severe liver disease in a dose-response pattern (adjusted hazard ratio for every 1 g/d increase 1.02; 95% CI, 1.01–1.02). No evidence of a threshold effect was found and risk was increased even in men who consumed less than 30 g of alcohol per day.[9] The incidence of chronic liver disease, cirrhosis, and hepatocellular carcinoma is expected to increase sharply in young adults in the near future. From a public health perspective, alcohol abuse and obesity should be addressed, and strategies designed to jointly reduce both alcohol consumption and obesity among adolescents are likely to produce much greater reductions in liver disease that strategies that address one condition alone.

Fetal alcohol spectrum disorder includes physical, mental, behavioral, and cognitive problems in infants with prenatal alcohol exposure. Alcohol is a teratogen with irreversible central nervous system effects. Prenatal alcohol exposure may result in structural birth defects including heart, kidney, eyes, and skeleton. The estimated global prevalence of fetal alcohol spectrum disorder in the general population of children ages 0 to 16.4 years was 7.7 per 1000 population. Fetal alcohol syndrome includes at least 2 of 3 characteristics: facial features, growth retardation, and clear evidence of brain involvement or neurobehavioral impairment. Early diagnosis is essential to provide education, anticipatory guidance, family support, and a medical home. The interventions should be individualized to patients' needs and may include occupational, speech, language, and behavior therapy and/or psychotropic pharmacotherapy.[10]

REFERENCES

1. Centers for Disease Control and Prevention (CDC). 1991-2015 high school youth risk behavior survey data. 2015. Available at: http://nccd.cdc.gov/youthonline/. Accessed October 6, 2018.

2. Skjakodegard HF, Danielsen YS, Morken M, et al. Study protocol: a randomized controlled trial evaluating the effect of family-based behavioral treatment of childhood and adolescent obesity-The FABO-study. BMC Public Health 2016;16(1):1106.

3. World Health Organization. Global status report on alcohol and health 2014. 2014.

4. Coley RL, Sims J, Carrano J. Environmental risks outweigh dopaminergic genetic risks for alcohol use and abuse from adolescence through early adulthood. Drug Alcohol Depend 2017;175:106–18.

5. Cohen E, Mackenzie RG, Yates GL. HEADSS, a psychosocial risk assessment instrument: implications for designing effective intervention programs for runaway youth. J Adolesc Health 1991;12(7):539–44.

6. Ewing JA. Detecting alcoholism: the cage questionnaire. JAMA 1984;252(14):1905–7.

7. Doycheva I, Watt KD, Rifai G, et al. Increasing burden of chronic liver disease among adolescents and young adults in the USA: a silent epidemic. Dig Dis Sci 2017;62(5):1373–80.

8. Alisi A, Nobili V. Metabolic syndrome and alcohol abuse: a potential hepatocarcinogenic mix in adolescents. Clin Gastroenterol Hepatol 2012;10(2):204 [author reply: 204–5].

9. Hagstrom H, Hemmingsson T, Discacciati A, et al. Alcohol consumption in late adolescence is associated with an increased risk of severe liver disease later in life. J Hepatol 2018;68(3):505–10.

10. Del Campo M, Jones KL. A review of the physical features of the fetal alcohol spectrum disorders. Eur J Med Genet 2017;60(1):55–64.

Alcohol Use Disorders in Alcoholic Liver Disease

Jessica L. Mellinger, MD, MSc[a],*, Gerald Scott Winder, MD, MSc[b]

KEYWORDS

- Alcohol dependence • Addiction • Biomarkers • Multidisciplinary care

KEY POINTS

- Alcohol use disorder (AUD) is a clinical diagnosis of harmful drinking characterized by loss of drinking control, severe drinking-related consequences, and impairment in multiple domains of life, tolerance to alcohol, and strong urges to drink.
- Diagnosis of AUD requires careful history taking and use of a nonjudgmental, open interpersonal style to establish and maintain a robust therapeutic alliance.
- Various psychotherapeutic and psychopharmacologic treatment options are available for AUD but are underutilized in alcoholic liver disease (ALD) for various reasons.
- The optimal treatment of ALD and AUD is multidisciplinary, though integrated care models are emerging and have not been systematically tested.

INTRODUCTION

Although many chronic medical diseases involve a complex interplay between biology and behavior, the cross-disciplinary pathophysiology of alcoholic liver disease (ALD) is particularly important because of concerning epidemiologic trends in alcohol use and ALD (see D. Axley, C. Taylor Richardson, and Ashwani K. Singal's article "Epidemiology of Alcohol Consumption and Societal Burden of Alcoholism and ALD," in this issue). Treating patients with ALD can be further complicated by some of the unfavorable effects of alcohol use disorders (AUDs) on the patient-provider alliance, patient support systems, and other general health behaviors as well as the stigma attached to both AUD and ALD. Awareness of and attention to these factors improves the ability of the medical provider to adequately care for patients with ALD. This article discusses the diagnosis and management of AUD, including unique aspects of the management of AUD in patients with ALD.

Disclosures: Dr Mellinger was funded by an AASLD (American Association for the Study of Liver Diseases) 2016 Clinical and Translational Research Award.
[a] Division of Gastroenterology and Hepatology, Michigan Medicine, 1500 East Medical Center Drive, SPC 5334, Ann Arbor, MI 48109, USA; [b] Department of Psychiatry, Michigan Medicine, 1500 East Medical Center Drive, SPC 5118, Ann Arbor, MI 48109, USA
* Corresponding author.
E-mail address: jmelling@med.umich.edu

Definition and Diagnosis of Alcohol Use, Misuse, and Disorders in Alcoholic Liver Disease

Diagnostic criteria and screening questionnaires

Despite logistic and attitudinal barriers to AUD diagnosis and management in the hepatology clinic, diagnosis is feasible and necessary. An AUD cannot be adequately treated without first being diagnosed. The most recent edition of the *Diagnostic and Statistical Manual of Mental Disorders* (*DSM*) Fifth Edition, defines AUD as mild, moderate, or severe based on the tally of negative consequences and symptoms.[1] These categories replaced prior *DSM-IV* categories of alcohol abuse and alcohol dependence.

Diagnosis begins with screening for alcohol use, a screening that usually occurs during the history-taking portion of the interview and can be uncomfortable and stigmatizing for patients, magnifying the importance of a working patient-provider alliance. Adopting a nonjudgmental, open, and accepting interview style can help maintain therapeutic alliance, which is a predictor of subsequent alcohol treatment success, even for nonpsychotherapists.[2] Patient engagement is key, as underreporting and denial of alcohol use is common, even in high-risk transplant patients and those enrolled in alcohol research studies.[3–5] Diagnosis is further complicated by the fact that symptoms of AUD and ALD may not be readily apparent, particularly in the early stages of ALD when drinking brings patients pleasure rather than feelings of illness. Patients are frequently unaware of what a standard serving of alcohol is, so providers should be able to educate patients about these serving sizes and adapt questioning accordingly (**Fig. 1**).

The content of the elicited social history should cover recent and remote drinking patterns (quantity and frequency), previous attempts to abstain, periods of prolonged

What Is a Standard Drink?

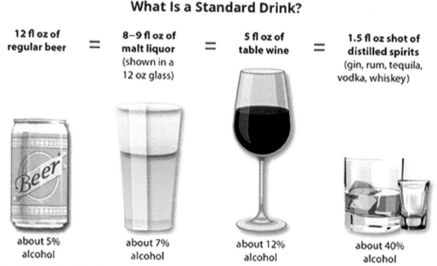

| **12 fl oz of regular beer** | = | **8–9 fl oz of malt liquor** (shown in a 12 oz glass) | = | **5 fl oz of table wine** | = | **1.5 fl oz shot of distilled spirits** (gin, rum, tequila, vodka, whiskey) |

| about 5% alcohol | about 7% alcohol | about 12% alcohol | about 40% alcohol |

Fig. 1. Standard drink measures in the United States. Each beverage portrayed represents one standard drink of pure alcohol, defined in the United States as 0.6 fl oz or 14 g. The percent of pure alcohol, expressed here as alcohol by volume, varies within and across beverage types. Although the standard drink amounts are helpful for following health guidelines, they may not reflect customary serving sizes. (*From* https://www.niaaa.nih.gov/alcohol-health/overview-alcohol-consumption/what-standard-drink. Accessed June 4, 2018.)

sobriety, negative effects of alcohol use, concurrent substance use (tobacco, illicit drugs, or marijuana), and perceptions and history of alcohol treatment. In advanced ALD (alcoholic cirrhosis and alcoholic hepatitis), a cognitive assessment is frequently essential given the effects of hepatic encephalopathy on AUD treatment planning, including patients' ability to engage in AUD treatment and retain what they learn. Two common, useful, and widely accepted screening tools for mental status in this regard are the Mini-Mental Status Examination and the Montreal Cognitive Assessment. Overt hepatic encephalopathy is often readily apparent by clinical history and examination while in-clinic screening for minimal hepatic encephalopathy can also be performed with a range of bedside techniques,[6] few of which have been tested in alcoholic cirrhosis patients with recent drinking. Best practices for interview-based assessment include expressing interest, empathy, and understanding as well as repairing any misalliance as it occurs.[2,7]

Every opportunity to identify and intervene in patients with AUD should be taken as screening leads to diagnosis and treatment. Regardless of location (clinic vs inpatient vs emergency department), screening is feasible and identifies patients with ALD in need of early intervention, particularly given that alcohol use is a common cofactor in injuries and hospital admissions.[8] Efforts to uncover alcohol use may be aided by use of structured, validated screening tools, such as the Alcohol Use Disorders Inventory Test (AUDIT),[9] a well-validated, highly sensitive and specific screening tool for alcohol use that also gives information on severity. Its original form includes 10 questions on consumption (questions 1–3), dependence symptoms (questions 4–6) and any alcohol-related problems (questions 7–10). Questions 1 to 3 are often used alone as the AUDIT-C as expedited screening for problem alcohol use.[10] AUDIT-C scores 4 to 5 or greater may indicate potential harmful alcohol use, whereas scores of 20 or greater on the full AUDIT may indicate alcohol dependence (now known as moderate/severe AUD).[10] Use of the AUDIT improves detection of alcohol use compared with hepatologist assessment alone, where it identified 22% more post-liver transplant patients as having consumed alcohol.[11] Consistent alcohol screening in all-comers to an inpatient general medicine ward was also shown to be feasible and effective in identifying heavy users, aided in ALD diagnosis, and improved connection to subsequent alcohol use treatment.[12] Importantly, the use of screening tools, such as AUDIT, has been shown to predict long-term clinical outcomes, including hospitalization for alcohol-related diagnoses, and may, when combined with feedback given to patients on the degree of their liver damage, be motivational for alcohol cessation.[13–15]

Alcohol biomarkers

Although screening questionnaires coupled with the history are helpful, patients are frequently less than candid about their alcohol use. This lack of candor is a particularly acute problem in the transplant setting where recent alcohol use may disqualify patients as candidates for a time. In earlier stages of ALD, lack of candor may mean a missed opportunity to diagnose and treat alcohol use and prevent progression to cirrhosis. Alcohol biomarkers are urine, blood, and hair testing that specifically identify alcohol use metabolites and give variable estimates of the time frame of recent drinking. Nonspecific laboratory testing, such as liver enzyme elevations, bilirubin elevation, gamma-glutamyl transferase (GGT), and the presence of a macrocytic anemia, may suggest alcohol use but on their own are inadequate to establish alcohol use in ALD because of the myriad other causes and contributors to their abnormality.[16] The use of alcohol biomarkers can be an aid to diagnosis and a therapeutic support for recovery but should not be used to catch or punish patients. The ideal way to integrate biomarkers into AUD treatment, however, is a subject in need of further study and consensus.

Discussing the use of alcohol biomarkers with patients *prior to* testing is critical in maintaining therapeutic alliance and improving alcohol use disclosure. The discussion itself can often precipitate meaningful candor about drinking, increasing the accuracy of drinking information and strengthening the patient-provider alliance. Patients should also be made aware of common environmental exposures that could trigger a positive result in some tests (ie, cold medicines, mouthwash, copious hand sanitizer, nonalcoholic beer, vanilla extract). Positive alcohol biomarker results are not evidence on their own of a disorder and should never be used in isolation to confirm or refute alcohol use but should be interpreted in the context of other laboratory testing, environmental exposure, physical examination, patient history, and the clinical interview. In this way, biomarker testing can be used as a catalyst for further conversation and connection to AUD treatment. *Providers choosing to use alcohol biomarkers in patients with ALD should be aware of the uses and limitations of this technology and should not base treatment decisions, particularly listing or delisting for transplant, solely on findings from biomarkers.*

Carbohydrate-deficient transferrin

Carbohydrate-deficient transferrin (CDT) is a measure of impaired transferrin glycosylation that results in CDT molecules in the presence of alcohol use. Typically reported as %CDT per total transferrin, to account for differences in total transferrin levels as a function of sex, weight, or other liver diseases, CDT has a half-life of 2 to 3 weeks.[17] Importantly, 60 g or more alcohol consumption is needed for CDT detection. Evidence suggests that increasing severity of liver disease can elevate %CDT levels in patients across liver disease causes and in the absence of alcohol use, indicating that caution is necessary in interpreting findings.[18–21] Some studies have found that combining CDT with GGT for alcohol-dependent patients improved test performance, though this study was not performed in patients with liver disease exclusively.[22]

Urinary ethyl glucuronide and ethyl sulfate

Alcohol is metabolized in the liver with most (>99%) metabolized via the well-known alcohol and acetaldehyde dehydrogenase pathways. However, a small (~0.1%) amount is metabolized by uridine 5'-diphospho- glucuronosyltransferase and sulfotransferase, producing ethyl glucuronide (EtG) and ethyl sulfate (EtS) resulting from the conjugation of ethanol with glucuronic acid in the liver.[23] Both are excreted in the urine but are also found in blood and hair. False positives can occur with exposure to alcohols in food (sauerkraut, mature bananas), cold medicines, mouthwash, and hand sanitizer.[23–25] False positives can be generated by the presence of endogenous alcohols from fermentation in diabetic patients with glycosuria and false negatives by bacterial contamination during a urinary tract infection. As a result, EtS is recommended to be paired as a confirmatory test because it is not affected by bacterial contamination.[23,26,27] Urine EtG/EtS have been studied in patients with liver disease, including those with cirrhosis; neither seems to be affected by advancing liver disease, though longer detection times for both EtG and EtS in renal failure have been seen.[28,29] In a study of urine EtG in patients with ALD before and after transplant, sensitivity and specificity for alcohol use detection were 89% and 99%, respectively, with urine EtG performing better than CDT alone or in combination with other markers of alcohol use (GGT, mean corpuscular volume).[30] Other studies in patients with a mixed cause of liver disease, including cirrhosis, found sensitivities of 76% and 82% for 3-day drinking detection for EtG and EtS, respectively, with higher specificities of 93% and 86%, respectively.[31] Hair EtG has been shown to detect moderate to heavy alcohol use (60 g of alcohol per day or more) when found at levels of 30 pg or higher[32,33] but may also have prolonged detection times similar to urinary EtG in patients with renal failure[34] and could be confounded by hair bleaching or dyeing.

Phosphatidylethanol

Phosphatidylethanol (PETH) is a phospholipid formed by the catalytic reaction of phosphatidylcholine and ethanol by phospholipase D occurring in the erythrocyte cell membrane.[35] A relatively new alcohol biomarker, PETH has a half-life of approximately 10 to 14 days, though this can be longer with more chronic, repeated heavy alcohol consumption[35–37] and does not seem to be influenced by age, body mass index, sex, kidney, or liver disease,[38–41] though women may have higher PETH levels for a given amount of alcohol consumption compared with men.[42] A single drink can be detectable for 12 days,[35] and the window of detection can extend out to 1 month. Although there are interindividual variations in PETH metabolism, PETH has been validated in a study of patients with chronic liver disease who had not undergone transplant at a cutoff of 80 ng/mL for 4 drinks per day or more with a sensitivity of 91% (95% confidence interval [CI], 82%–100%) and a specificity of 77% (95% CI, 70%–83%).[41] Another study of PETH used in both pre- and post-ALD transplant patients revealed a sensitivity of 100% (79%–100%) and a specificity of 96% (91%–99%).[43] PETH is useful for determining if any alcohol intake occurred, but because of individual variation in both metabolism and pharmacokinetics of PETH degradation, it may be less useful for truly quantifying the amount of alcohol used in a given time frame.[36] Further research to clearly establish cutoffs in patients with liver disease, verify time windows for detection, and confirm any possible false-positive effects of phospholipase D activity in patients with liver disease is needed.[44]

Management: Helping Patients Achieve and Maintain Abstinence

The experience of medical providers caring for patients with alcohol use disorder

Hepatology and primary care providers are often challenged in caring for patients with ALD and may feel that their options for meaningful intervention are few. However, one of the most powerful predictors of better outcomes in AUD treatment is the quality of the therapeutic relationship they form with their patients. The therapeutic alliance between patient and provider has been defined in multiple ways according to different theories and disciplines throughout medicine and mental health.[45,46] This alliance influences the outcomes of AUD treatment[47] particularly when patients may have lower levels of motivation or self-efficacy.[48] We can infer that the therapeutic alliance between patients with ALD and their hepatology provider is likely of similar importance to the medical treatment of patients with ALD, particularly given that patients with ALD report listening to and trusting their medical providers.[49] Hepatology providers may not be familiar with or attend to the details of a therapeutic alliance (**Table 1**). Yet aspects of AUD's signs and symptoms and its stigma may impact the quality of the alliance and clinical outcomes, requiring ongoing effort to maintain good working relationships with patients.

The need for multidisciplinary care of patients with alcohol use disorder and alcoholic liver disease

AUD and ALD disease processes overlap, but expertise in treating both conditions rarely does on the level of individual clinics or providers. As a consequence, patients with ALD often fall through the cracks and fail to obtain the full range of treatment options for both AUD and ALD. Particularly in more advanced AUD, whereby brief interventions may be less effective, referral to expert substance use treatment is recommended. Despite the inherent challenges in establishing such collaborations, the importance of establishing reciprocal consultative relationships between hepatology

Table 1
Components of a high-quality therapeutic alliance

The 6 C's of a Patient-Provider Alliance	
Choice	Patients desire a choice about who they see and where. Implicit to informed consent, they want a choice among recommended treatments, including alternatives.
Competence	Patients expect their physician to have a robust knowledge base; good technical repertoire of diagnosis and treatment; sound clinical judgment; and awareness of one's limitations, scope of practice, and need to refer.
Communication	Patients have the ability to describe their symptoms; when this might be difficult, providers facilitate needed communication. Providers respond to patients' preferences about what they want to know and in a way suited to their needs and values. When conflict arises, good communication prevents escalation.
Compassion	Along with their desire for technical medical proficiency, patients desire support and compassion in their time of need. This support may consist of reinforcing patients' existing values, feelings, or experiences but also might entail some level of guided and empathic reconsideration and reevaluation of such.
Continuity	The investment of time on the part of physician and patients to build a durable and trusting relationship that extends over time. Relationships of this kind are more efficient and hold the potential to facilitate greater adherence and behavior changes.
(No) Conflict of interest	A physician's primary concern is patients' well-being. A physician's care of patients takes precedence over the physician's personal interests, especially financial interests.

Data from Emanuel EJ, Dubler NN. Preserving the physician-patient relationship in the era of managed care. JAMA 1995;273(4):326.

and mental health cannot be overstated when discussing optimal ALD management strategies. Without access to AUD experts as well as facing provider or system-level triage and referral barriers, medical providers may conclude that AUDs are simply outside of their scope of practice and avoid regularly asking about drinking or using biomarkers to detect it. Furthermore, in a busy liver clinic, there may not be consensus among providers, adequate financial incentives, or feasible logistics to take on the extra effort of AUD diagnosis and management. Until more collaborative AUD and ALD treatment models have been broadly established and tested, it is important for medical providers to be aware of and prepare for these stark inevitabilities.

Alcohol cessation: what a medical provider can do in the clinic

There is abundant evidence that ongoing alcohol use, particularly in the setting of advanced ALD (alcoholic cirrhosis [AC] and alcoholic hepatitis [AH]), results in worse outcomes, including increased rates of variceal bleeding, ascites, hepatic encephalopathy, and death.[50,51] In the posttransplant setting, recurrent AC results from severe AUD relapse and may progress more rapidly, with the graft becoming cirrhotic in as little as 5 years.[52] In less advanced stages (alcohol-related steatosis or fibrosis), complete alcohol cessation may result in improvement and regression of steatosis and fibrosis.[53] *As a result, all patients with ALD should be advised to abstain completely from alcohol use.* Patients with comorbid viral hepatitis, including hepatitis C, should also abstain from all alcohol use given the accelerated liver damage and increased liver cancer risk that can occur in the setting of ALD and HCV.[54]

Once ALD has been diagnosed and the degree of alcohol misuse has been character-ized, referral to alcohol treatment, particularly in patients with moderate to severe AUD or advanced AC/AH, is mandatory. Screening and brief intervention is generally accepted as more effective for less severe alcohol misuse and is unlikely to be effective for more severe AUDs, whereby referral to alcohol use treatment is necessary.[55] Given the frequency of psychiatric comorbidities occurring with AUDs (such as depression and anxiety), many patients will benefit from seeing a mental health provider. Yet many are reluctant to accept such a referral. Hepatology clinics rarely have direct affiliation with addiction providers, and specialized care referrals to another site may result in poor follow-up. Without direct consultation with liver specialists, and facing medically ill pa-tients with advanced liver disease, mental health specialists may defer pharmacologic treatments that might otherwise benefit patients when weighing potential medication side effects against the liver damage of ongoing drinking.

For medical providers faced with patients reluctant to stop drinking and engage in AUD treatment, motivational interviewing (MI) may be helpful (**Table 2**). In patients ambivalent about alcohol cessation, MI has been shown to be helpful in resolving ambivalence and helping patients change behaviors[56] but is not a skill set common

Table 2	
Components of motivational interviewing	
4 Key Elements of the Spirit of MI	
Partnership	MI is done for and with patients rather than to them. It entails seeing their life and circumstances through their eyes. Because patients are experts on themselves, the clinician activates patients' intrinsic self-knowledge and initiative in the service of change. A helpful analogy is that partnering with patients in MI has more in common with the grace and choreography of a ballroom dance with them rather than the tension and confrontation of a wrestling match. Partnering also requires that a clinician have self-awareness about his or her own agenda and aspirations that may differ from the patients'.
Acceptance	The clinician disregards his or her personal approval or disapproval and profoundly accepts patients. Acceptance in MI invokes the work of Carl Rogers, which includes 4 elements: • Absolute worth, also termed unconditional positive regard: It is the idea that, paradoxically, when people are accepted as they are, they are freed to change. • Autonomy support: Recognizing patients' freedom of choice reduces defensiveness and facilitates change. • Affirmation: It is seeking and acknowledging patients' efforts and strengths. • Accurate empathy: It is an active interest in and effort toward seeing the world through patients' eyes.
Compassion	In MI, compassion is defined as the active promotion of and the deliberate commitment to the patients' welfare, giving priority to their needs and eschewing exploitation.
Evocation	Much of what is done in medicine is concerned with what is wrong or where there is a deficit. When this is found, the remedy is provided by the clinician. This paradigm is less helpful in behavior change. Emphasizing the patients' extant strengths and values, the clinician evokes the patients' *own* internal ambivalence about what to do and facilitates patients working toward its resolution.

Data from Winder GS, Mellinger J, Fontana RJ. Preventing drinking relapse in patients with alco-holic liver disease: your role is essential in preventing, detecting, and co-managing alcoholic liver disease in inpatient and ambulatory settings. Current Psychiatry 2015;14(12):22–32.

in hepatology clinic providers and may be difficult to deploy in a busy liver clinic with highly medically complex patients. Nonetheless, training to incorporate MI into medical practice is available via the Motivational Interviewing Network of Trainers (www. motivationalinterviewing.org).

Psychosocial and behavioral approaches to alcohol use disorder treatment in patients with alcoholic liver disease

There are a wide variety of AUD treatment modalities available to patients, though relatively few have been studied exclusively in patients with ALD. Major categories of treatment include inpatient alcohol rehabilitation, group therapies, one-on-one therapies, family/couples counseling, mutual aid societies (such Alcoholics Anonymous and others), and relapse prevention medications. Within therapists' repertoires are various paradigms and modalities of psychotherapy that target different mechanisms of behavior change. These modalities include cognitive-behavior therapy (CBT), MI, motivational enhancement therapy (MET), contingency management, 12-step facilitation, network therapy, and couples/family counseling. However, there have been little data to show that one treatment modality is consistently superior to another across all categories of populations.[57] The choice of modality, intensity, and duration of behavioral interventions is variable and best determined by the addiction professional after initial assessment in conjunction with patient preferences and abilities. The American Society of Addiction Medicine suggests a tiered approach to treatment based on severity of alcohol misuse. For those with more severe AUD (moderate to severe), which includes many if not most patients with advanced ALD, concurrent behavioral and pharmacologic treatment may be necessary with brief interventions less likely to produce long-term alcohol cessation.[55]

There have been several small studies of psychosocial treatments in patients with ALD. A recent systematic review of psychosocial treatment trials in ALD found that integrating AUD treatment in the medical clinic alongside liver disease treatment produced better abstinence rates than usual care, which was most often a referral to an unaffiliated alcohol treatment provider.[58] Types of AUD treatment evaluated in both randomized and observational trials include CBT, MET, psychoeducation, and MI, with modalities combined in varying ways in each trial. Five randomized controlled trials were reported, 3 of which enrolled AC exclusively and only one of which showed a statistically significant benefit with an integrated intervention combining CBT and MET with medical care.[59] Other observational studies evaluated psychosocial interventions for patients with hepatitis C with alcohol use[58] and showed modest improvement in alcohol abstinence. Based on these findings, integrated, multidisciplinary care remains the best option for managing advanced ALD (AC and AH) and AUD, though it may not be practical in all care delivery settings and needs further study.

Relapse prevention medications

Pharmacotherapy for alcohol use includes both Food and Drug Administration (FDA)– and non-FDA– approved medications (**Table 3**). There are 3 FDA-approved AUD medications: disulfiram, naltrexone, and acamprosate. Disulfiram inhibits acetaldehyde dehydrogenase, resulting in accumulation of acetaldehyde, which produces noxious physical symptoms in the presence of alcohol. Use in patients with established ALD is contraindicated given that it is metabolized by the liver and has well-established hepatotoxicity, including instances of acute liver failure. Naltrexone and acamprosate are more commonly used in the general AUD population. Naltrexone, a mu-opioid receptor antagonist, has been shown to be effective in alcohol reduction and cessation in the general population[60,61], but its use has been limited in patients with ALD

Table 3
Alcohol relapse prevention medications in ALD

Drug	Mechanism of Action	Dose	Metabolism	Excretion	Considerations in ALD
Naltrexone[a]	Opioid receptor antagonist	50 mg daily orally or 380 mg subcutaneous monthly	Hepatic	Mostly renal, fecal 2–3%	Not studied in ALD patients Hepatotoxicity concerns
Acamprosate[a]	NMDA receptor antagonist	666 mg 3 times daily	None	Renal	Unstudied in ALD patients but no reported instances of hepatotoxicity.
Gabapentin	Modulates GABA activity via presynaptic calcium channels	600–1800 mg daily	None	Renal 75%, fecal 25%	Unstudied in ALD patients Monitor closely for renal dysfunction and worsening mental status/sedation
Baclofen	GABA-B receptor agonist	30–60 mg daily in 3 divided doses	Limited hepatic	Renal	Single RCT in ALD patients showed benefit at dose of 10 mg three times daily
Topiramate	Augments GABA activity, glutamate antagonist	75–400 mg daily	Not extensively metabolized	Renal	Unstudied in ALD patients.

[a] Approved by FDA for AUD treatment. Disulfiram is not included on this list because it is not recommended for use in ALD patients.
Data from Winder GS, Mellinger J, Fontana RJ. Preventing drinking relapse in patients with alcoholic liver disease: your role is essential in preventing, detecting, and co-managing alcoholic liver disease in inpatient and ambulatory settings. Current Psychiatry 2015;14(12):22–8.

because of hepatic metabolism and concerns about hepatotoxicity. Hepatotoxicity with naltrexone has been shown in as many as 30% of patients and to be dose dependent with some laboratory abnormalities resolving with ongoing therapy. One study showed hepatotoxicity in a minority of patients at doses of 300 mg daily.[62] Other studies have not shown elevated hepatotoxicity in the treatment group.[63] Depot injections of naltrexone may have a more favorable side effect profile given their bypass of first-pass metabolism though neither oral nor depot formulations have been tested in patients with liver disease, including ALD. Caution is also warranted with the use of naltrexone or other opioid receptor antagonists, such as nalmefene, given their interference with opioid medications that are widely prescribed in the general population as well as in patients with ALD. Were naltrexone to be used for relapse prevention, a 7- to 10-day opioid washout period is advised.

Acamprosate, an N-methyl-D-aspartate receptor antagonist, has minimal hepatic metabolism and has not been associated with clinically apparent liver injury. It has been extensively studied in the general alcohol use population but not in patients with ALD specifically. Two recent meta-analyses showed a modest effect on return to drinking for acamprosate in those with problem alcohol use, with the Jonas and colleagues[61] meta-analysis reporting a number-needed-to-treat (NNT) of 12 (95% CI 8–26) for acamprosate and NNT of 20 (95% CI 11–500) for naltrexone 50 mg orally.[60] Although none of these FDA-approved medications have been tested specifically in patients with ALD, acamprosate is generally thought to be safe for use even in advanced liver disease because of the absence of hepatic metabolism and few reports of liver-related toxicity. Acamprosate is metabolized by the kidney so dose reduction or cessation may be necessary in patients with renal disease. When comparing different clinical alcohol use outcomes (ie, reducing heavy drinking vs promoting full abstinence), acamprosate was shown to have a larger effect size in maintaining abstinence, whereas naltrexone showed more effective reduction of heavy drinking and craving.[64]

Several medications have been shown to have some benefit in relapse prevention but have not been FDA approved for AUD treatment. Baclofen, a γ-aminobutyric acid (GABA)-B receptor agonist, is the only AUD pharmacotherapy option to have been tested in a randomized controlled fashion in patients with AC alcoholic cirrhosis with comorbid AUD. In a small randomized trial of both compensated and decompensated alcoholic cirrhotic patients, a 12-week course of baclofen 10 mg three times daily had an acceptable safety profile and resulted in improved rates of total alcohol abstinence and decreased relapse compared with controls.[65] Notably, however, patients with hepatic encephalopathy were excluded from this trial. Gabapentin, an anticonvulsant that modulates GABA activity, is approved for epileptic seizures and neuropathic pain. In one randomized placebo-controlled trial, it was shown to improve rates of total abstinence as well as decreased heavy drinking days, decreases in alcohol craving, and improved sleep at a dose of 1800 mg daily (600 mg 3 times daily).[66] Gabapentin has minimal hepatic metabolism and is renally excreted. Although there are no specific data in patients with ALD, there have been few reports of hepatotoxicity and no reported cases of acute liver failure or chronic liver injury described. Other medications that have been used off label in small studies of non-ALD patients include topiramate,[67,68] ondansetron,[69] and varenicline[70], but none are approved for AUD treatment and none have been tested in patients with ALD. Although hepatic metabolism of FDA- and non-FDA–approved pharmacotherapy for AUDs is variable, most are excreted renally, which should be kept in mind when prescribing in patients with AC and AH, given the high degree of comorbid kidney injury in this population.

Special considerations in patients with alcoholic liver disease
Patients with ALD seeking AUD therapy will encounter unique challenges. Physical stigmata of advanced cirrhosis or AH may impact their willingness to engage in group therapy given concerns about their appearance and the perceptions of others. These patients have a high burden of medical visits complicating their ability to adhere to an outpatient regimen of therapy and/or support group visits. For patients with ALD needing intensive outpatient (IOP) or inpatient residential rehabilitation, their medical visits and medical complexity can both affect their ability to even make it to treatment appointments and, once there, may affect their ability to meaningfully participate in cognitively demanding extended therapy sessions. Hepatic encephalopathy, along with myriad other physical challenges of decompensated cirrhosis, will challenge patients' ability to engage in treatment, particularly because long periods of sitting and attention are required in IOP or intensive inpatient rehabilitation. In patients who are actively drinking, providers should be aware of the possibility of alcohol withdrawal in already medically complex patients and consider inpatient admission for treatment, alcohol detoxification, and stabilization.

SUMMARY

Although technically outside the training of medical providers, those caring for patients with ALD will benefit from education on the broad array of alcohol use treatment options available in order to facilitate proactive and knowledgeable discussion about AUD treatment with patients with ALD. AUD treatment discussions that originate from the medical provider of patients with ALD may aid in receptivity and bridging to professional substance use disorder treatment referrals by capitalizing on existing clinical rapport and alliance, overcoming misconceptions about effectiveness and availability of alcohol use treatment modalities, and linking the biological and behavioral aspects of the disease.

REFERENCES

1. American Psychiatric Association. Diagnostic and statistical manual of mental disorders (DSM-5®). Arlington (VA): American Psychiatric Publishing; 2013.
2. Rosenthal RN, Ries RK, Zweben JE. Medical management techniques and collaborative care: integrating behavioral with pharmacologic interventions in addiction treatment. In: Ries RK, Fiellin DA, Miller SC, et al, editors. The ASAM principles of addiction medicine. 5th edition. Philadelphia (PA): Wolters Kluwer Health; 2014. p. 1008–20.
3. Webzell I, Ball D, Bell J, et al. Substance use by liver transplant candidates: an anonymous urinalysis study. Liver Transpl 2011;17(10):1200–4.
4. Fleming MF, Smith MJ, Oslakovic E, et al. Phosphatidylethanol detects moderate-to-heavy alcohol use in liver transplant recipients. Alcohol Clin Exp Res 2017; 41(4):857–62.
5. McCaul ME, Wand GS. Detecting deception in our research participants: are your participants who you think they are? Alcohol Clin Exp Res 2018;42(2):230–7.
6. Tapper EB, Parikh ND, Waljee AK, et al. Diagnosis of minimal hepatic encephalopathy: a systematic review of point-of-care diagnostic tests. Am J Gastroenterol 2018;113(4):529–38.
7. Ries RK, Fiellin DA, Miller SC, et al. The ASAM principles of addiction medicine. 5th edition. Philadelphia: Wolters Kluwer Health; 2014.
8. Cherpitel CJ, Ye Y, Bond J, et al. Multi-level analysis of alcohol-related injury among emergency department patients: a cross-national study. Addiction 2005;100(12):1840–50.

9. Conigrave KM, Hall WD, Saunders JB. The AUDIT questionnaire: choosing a cut-off score. Alcohol use disorder identification test. Addiction 1995;90(10):1349–56.

10. Bradley KA, DeBenedetti AF, Volk RJ, et al. AUDIT-C as a brief screen for alcohol misuse in primary care. Alcohol Clin Exp Res 2007;31(7):1208–17.

11. Donnadieu-Rigole H, Olive L, Nalpas B, et al. Follow-up of alcohol consumption after liver transplantation: interest of an addiction team? Alcohol Clin Exp Res 2017;41(1):165–70.

12. Westwood G, Meredith P, Atkins S, et al. Universal screening for alcohol misuse in acute medical admissions is feasible and identifies patients at high risk of liver disease. J Hepatol 2017;67(3):559–67.

13. Au DH, Kivlahan DR, Bryson CL, et al. Alcohol screening scores and risk of hospitalizations for GI conditions in men. Alcohol Clin Exp Res 2007;31(3):443–51.

14. Sheron N. Alcohol and liver disease in Europe–Simple measures have the potential to prevent tens of thousands of premature deaths. J Hepatol 2016;64(4): 957–67.

15. Sheron N, Moore M, O'Brien W, et al. Feasibility of detection and intervention for alcohol-related liver disease in the community: the Alcohol and Liver Disease Detection study (ALDDeS). Br J Gen Pract 2013;63(615):e698–705.

16. Litten RZ, Bradley AM, Moss HB. Alcohol biomarkers in applied settings: recent advances and future research opportunities. Alcohol Clin Exp Res 2010;34(6): 955–67.

17. Fagan KJ, Irvine KM, McWhinney BC, et al. BMI but not stage or etiology of nonalcoholic liver disease affects the diagnostic utility of carbohydrate-deficient transferrin. Alcohol Clin Exp Res 2013;37(10):1771–8.

18. DiMartini A, Day N, Lane T, et al. Carbohydrate deficient transferrin in abstaining patients with end-stage liver disease. Alcohol Clin Exp Res 2001;25(12):1729–33.

19. Allen JP, Wurst FM, Thon N, et al. Assessing the drinking status of liver transplant patients with alcoholic liver disease. Liver Transpl 2013;19(4):369–76.

20. Stewart SH, Reuben A, Anton RF. Relationship of abnormal chromatographic pattern for carbohydrate-deficient transferrin with severe liver disease. Alcohol Alcohol 2017;52(1):24–8.

21. Verbeek J, Crunelle CL, Leurquin-Sterk G, et al. Ethyl glucuronide in hair is an accurate biomarker of chronic excessive alcohol use in patients with alcoholic cirrhosis. Clin Gastroenterol Hepatol 2018;16(3):454–6.

22. Anton RF, Lieber C, Tabakoff B, CDTect Study Group. Carbohydrate-deficient transferrin and gamma-glutamyltransferase for the detection and monitoring of alcohol use: results from a multisite study. Alcohol Clin Exp Res 2002;26(8): 1215–22.

23. Walsham NE, Sherwood RA. Ethyl glucuronide. Ann Clin Biochem 2012;49(2): 110–7.

24. Reisfield GM, Goldberger BA, Pesce AJ, et al. Ethyl glucuronide, ethyl sulfate, and ethanol in urine after intensive exposure to high ethanol content mouthwash. J Analytical Toxicol 2011;35(5):264–8.

25. Reisfield GM, Goldberger BA, Crews BO, et al. Ethyl glucuronide, ethyl sulfate, and ethanol in urine after sustained exposure to an ethanol-based hand sanitizer. J Analytical Toxicol 2011;35(2):85–91.

26. Helander A, Olsson I, Dahl H. Postcollection synthesis of ethyl glucuronide by bacteria in urine may cause false identification of alcohol consumption. Clin Chem 2007;53(10):1855–7.

27. Helander A, Beck O. Ethyl sulfate: a metabolite of ethanol in humans and a potential biomarker of acute alcohol intake. J Anal Toxicol 2005;29(5):270–4.

28. Wurst FM, Dresen S, Allen JP, et al. Ethyl sulphate: a direct ethanol metabolite reflecting recent alcohol consumption. Addiction 2006;101(2):204–11.
29. Høiseth G, Nordal K, Pettersen E, et al. Prolonged urinary detection times of EtG and EtS in patients with decreased renal function. Alcohol Clin Exp Res 2012; 36(7):1148–51.
30. Staufer K, Andresen H, Vettorazzi E, et al. Urinary ethyl glucuronide as a novel screening tool in patients pre- and post-liver transplantation improves detection of alcohol consumption. Hepatology 2011;54(5):1640–9.
31. Stewart SH, Koch DG, Burgess DM, et al. Sensitivity and specificity of urinary ethyl glucuronide and ethyl sulfate in liver disease patients. Alcohol Clin Exp Res 2013;37(1):150–5.
32. Stewart SH, Koch DG, Willner IR, et al. Hair ethyl glucuronide is highly sensitive and specific for detecting moderate-to-heavy drinking in patients with liver disease. Alcohol Alcohol 2013;48(1):83–7.
33. Sterneck M, Yegles M, Rothkirch von G, et al. Determination of ethyl glucuronide in hair improves evaluation of long-term alcohol abstention in liver transplant candidates. Liver Int 2014;34(3):469–76.
34. Høiseth G, Morini L, Ganss R, et al. Higher levels of hair ethyl glucuronide in patients with decreased kidney function. Alcohol Clin Exp Res 2013;37(Suppl 1): E14–6.
35. Nguyen VL, Haber PS, Seth D. Applications and challenges for the use of phosphatidylethanol testing in liver disease patients (mini review). Alcohol Clin Exp Res 2018;42(2):238–43.
36. Gnann H, Weinmann W, Thierauf A. Formation of phosphatidylethanol and its subsequent elimination during an extensive drinking experiment over 5 days. Alcohol Clin Exp Res 2012;36(9):1507–11.
37. Schröck A, Wurst FM, Thon N, et al. Assessing phosphatidylethanol (PEth) levels reflecting different drinking habits in comparison to the alcohol use disorders identification test - C (AUDIT-C). Drug Alcohol Depend 2017;178:80–6.
38. Wurst FM, Thon N, Aradottir S, et al. Phosphatidylethanol: normalization during detoxification, gender aspects and correlation with other biomarkers and self-reports. Addict Biol 2010;15(1):88–95.
39. Viel G, Boscolo-Berto R, Cecchetto G, et al. Phosphatidylethanol in blood as a marker of chronic alcohol use: a systematic review and meta-analysis. Int J Mol Sci 2012;13(11):14788–812.
40. Stewart SH, Reuben A, Brzezinski WA, et al. Preliminary evaluation of phosphatidylethanol and alcohol consumption in patients with liver disease and hypertension. Alcohol Alcohol 2009;44(5):464–7.
41. Stewart SH, Koch DG, Willner IR, et al. Validation of blood phosphatidylethanol as an alcohol consumption biomarker in patients with chronic liver disease. Alcohol Clin Exp Res 2014;38(6):1706–11.
42. Simon TW. Providing context for phosphatidylethanol as a biomarker of alcohol consumption with a pharmacokinetic model. Regul Toxicol Pharmacol 2018;94: 163–71.
43. Andresen-Streichert H, Beres Y, Weinmann W, et al. Improved detection of alcohol consumption using the novel marker phosphatidylethanol in the transplant setting: results of a prospective study. Transpl Int 2017;30(6):611–20.
44. Nguyen VL, Paull P, Haber PS, et al. Evaluation of a novel method for the analysis of alcohol biomarkers: ethyl glucuronide, ethyl sulfate and phosphatidylethanol. Alcohol 2018;67:7–13.

45. Emanuel EJ, Dubler NN. Preserving the physician-patient relationship in the era of managed care. JAMA 1995;273(4):323–9.

46. Horvath AO, Symonds BD. Relation between working alliance and outcome in psychotherapy: a meta-analysis. J Couns Psychol 1991;38(2):139–49.

47. Connors GJ, Carroll KM, DiClemente CC, et al. The therapeutic alliance and its relationship to alcoholism treatment participation and outcome. J Consult Clin Psychol 1997;65(4):588–98.

48. Ilgen MA, McKellar J, Moos R, et al. Therapeutic alliance and the relationship between motivation and treatment outcomes in patients with alcohol use disorder. J Subst Abuse Treat 2006;31(2):157–62.

49. Mellinger JL, Scott Winder G, DeJonckheere M, et al. Misconceptions, preferences and barriers to alcohol use disorder treatment in alcohol-related cirrhosis. J Subst Abuse Treat 2018;91:20–7.

50. Lucey MR, Connor JT, Boyer TD, et al, DIVERT Study Group. Alcohol consumption by cirrhotic subjects: patterns of use and effects on liver function. Am J Gastroenterol 2008;103(7):1698–706.

51. Louvet A, Labreuche J, Artru F, et al. Drivers of short- and long-term mortality in severe alcoholic hepatitis: a complex relationship between alcohol relapse and early improvement in liver function. Hepatology 2016;64:22A.

52. Dumortier JEROM, Dharancy SEB, Cannesson AEL, et al. Recurrent alcoholic cirrhosis in severe alcoholic relapse after liver transplantation: a frequent and serious complication. Am J Gastroenterol 2015;110(8):1–7.

53. Thiele M, Rausch V, Fluhr G, et al. Controlled attenuation parameter and alcoholic hepatic steatosis: diagnostic accuracy and role of alcohol detoxification. J Hepatol 2018;68(5):1025–32.

54. Alavi M, Janjua NZ, Chong M, et al. The contribution of alcohol use disorder to decompensated cirrhosis among people with hepatitis C: an international study. J Hepatol 2018;68(3):393–401.

55. Jonas DE, Garbutt JC, Amick HR, et al. Behavioral counseling after screening for alcohol misuse in primary care: a systematic review and meta-analysis for the U.S. Preventive Services Task Force. Ann Intern Med 2012;157(9):645–54.

56. Miller WR, Rollnick S. Motivational interviewing. 3rd edition. New York: Guilford Press; 2012.

57. Klimas J, Tobin H, Field C-A, et al. Psychosocial interventions to reduce alcohol consumption in concurrent problem alcohol and illicit drug users. Cochrane Database Syst Rev 2014;(12):CD009269.

58. Khan A, Tansel A, White DL, et al. Efficacy of Psychosocial interventions in inducing and maintaining alcohol abstinence in patients with chronic liver disease: a systematic review. Clin Gastroenterol Hepatol 2016;14(2):191–202.e1-4.

59. Willenbring ML, Olson DH. A randomized trial of integrated outpatient treatment for medically ill alcoholic men. Arch Intern Med 1999;159(16):1946–52.

60. Donoghue K, Elzerbi C, Saunders R, et al. The efficacy of acamprosate and naltrexone in the treatment of alcohol dependence, Europe versus the rest of the world: a meta-analysis. Addiction 2015;110(6):920–30.

61. Jonas DE, Amick HR, Feltner C, et al. Pharmacotherapy for adults with alcohol use disorders in outpatient settings: a systematic review and meta-analysis. JAMA 2014;311(18):1889–900.

62. Mitchell JE. Naltrexone and hepatotoxicity. Lancet 1986;1(8491):1215.

63. Croop RS, Faulkner EB, Labriola DF. The safety profile of naltrexone in the treatment of alcoholism. Results from a multicenter usage study. The Naltrexone Usage Study Group. Arch Gen Psychiatry 1997;54(12):1130–5.

64. Maisel NC, Blodgett JC, Wilbourne PL, et al. Meta-analysis of naltrexone and acamprosate for treating alcohol use disorders: when are these medications most helpful? Addiction 2013;108(2):275–93.
65. Addolorato G, Leggio L, Ferrulli A, et al. Effectiveness and safety of baclofen for maintenance of alcohol abstinence in alcohol-dependent patients with liver cirrhosis: randomised, double-blind controlled study. Lancet 2007;370(9603): 1915–22.
66. Mason BJ, Quello S, Goodell V, et al. Gabapentin treatment for alcohol dependence: a randomized clinical trial. JAMA Intern Med 2014;174(1):70–7.
67. Johnson BA, Ait-Daoud N, Bowden CL, et al. Oral topiramate for treatment of alcohol dependence: a randomised controlled trial. Lancet 2003;361(9370): 1677–85.
68. Johnson BA, Rosenthal N, Capece JA, et al. Topiramate for treating alcohol dependence: a randomized controlled trial. JAMA 2007;298(14):1641–51.
69. Johnson BA, Roache JD, Javors MA, et al. Ondansetron for reduction of drinking among biologically predisposed alcoholic patients: a randomized controlled trial. JAMA 2000;284(8):963–71.
70. de Bejczy A, Löf E, Walther L, et al. Varenicline for treatment of alcohol dependence: a randomized, placebo-controlled trial. Alcohol Clin Exp Res 2015; 39(11):2189–99.

Pathogenesis of Alcoholic Liver Disease: An Update

Themistoklis Kourkoumpetis, MD[a], Gagan Sood, MD[b],*

KEYWORDS

- Pathogenesis • Alcohol • Alcoholism • Liver • Microbiome • Mycobiome
- Acetaldehyde • Toxicity

KEY POINTS

- Chronic alcohol consumption leads to fat accumulation and alcoholic fatty liver disease, which sometimes leads to alcoholic steatohepatitis.
- The splice variant of HSD17B13 encodes the hepatic lipid droplet protein hydroxysteroid 17-beta dehydrogenase-13 and is associated with 42% decreased risk of alcoholic liver disease (ALD).
- Alcohol can lead to fungal and bacterial dysbiosis, which in turn can alter intestinal inflammation, permeability, and substrate availability to Kupffer cells and the hepatic parenchyma.
- Pilot findings show that stool transplantation or probiotics seem to reverse dysbiosis and improve outcomes of severe alcoholic hepatitis.
- Environmental pollution is an underexplored field of alcoholic liver disease pathogenesis that may play a crucial role in ALD.

INTRODUCTION

Alcohol abuse is the seventh leading risk factor for death and disability-adjusted life-years globally and the first cause of death among people between 15 to 49 years of age.[1] Complications of ethanol differ; not all individuals who abuse alcohol go on to develop cirrhosis or alcoholic hepatitis. This observation may be related to differences in human alcohol metabolism and differences in gender, genetic and environmental factors, diet, and microbiome.

Upon its ingestion, ethanol comes in contact with the gastric mucosa, where it undergoes its first-pass metabolism into acetaldehyde. When ingested with a meal, ethanol's gastric absorption rates have been reported to fluctuate from 30% to 100% among healthy individuals, with only a small amount transitioning to the distal small

The authors have nothing to disclose.
[a] Department of Gastroenterology, Baylor College of Medicine, 6620 Main Street, Suite 1450, Houston, TX 77030, USA; [b] Department of Surgery, Division of Abdominal Transplantation, Baylor College of Medicine, 6620 Main Street, Suite 1450, Houston, TX 77030, USA
* Corresponding author.
E-mail address: gksood@bcm.edu

intestine.[2,3] Further transition of ethanol into the small and large intestine results in its metabolism by the microbiome. Along the way, ethanol becomes bioavailable through its rapid transit into the portal system through the gastric and small intestinal mucosa. Duration and amount of ethanol ingestion result in variable changes in the body's ability to metabolize it, resulting in progressive hepatotoxicity through the production of acetaldehyde in hepatocytes, gastric mucosal cells and by intestinal bacteria. The interaction between the microbiome and the host's liver is of particular interest in alcoholic liver disease (ALD), where alcohol has been shown to both change the composition of the microbiome and impair intestinal integrity and barrier function. Further microbiome changes seem to play a role in the leakage of lipopolysaccharide from gram-negative bacteria into the portal circulation, further activating Kupffer cells that initiate and sustain subsequent inflammatory responses. Activation of Kupffer cells is a central element in the pathogenesis of ALD. Kupffer cells in the liver are activated by bacterial endotoxin (lipopolysaccharide-LPS) through Toll-like receptor 4 (TLR4), and the level of LPS is increased in the portal and the systemic circulations after excessive alcohol intake. These observations suggest that gut-derived LPS is a central mediator of inflammation in alcoholic steatohepatitis. Microbiome manipulation shows promise in preventing alcohol-related hepatic changes. Further research is needed to establish specific treatment targets.

THE SPECTRUM OF ALCOHOLIC LIVER DISEASE

Light-to-moderate consumption of alcohol is defined as up to 1 drink per day for women and up to 2 drinks per day for men; these amounts are considered safe. Excessive drinking can lead to a spectrum of ALD. The first step is progressive fat accumulation leading to alcoholic fatty liver disease (AFLD). This accumulation is not always followed by inflammation or progression to alcoholic steatohepatitis (ASH). ASH develops in one-third of patients with AFLD and about one-tenth of them go on to develop cirrhosis.[4]

ETHANOL METABOLISM IN THE HEPATOCYTE

Ethanol's hepatotoxicity is mainly mediated through its conversion to acetaldehyde.

There are 3 classic main hepatocyte pathways of ethanol metabolism that lead to the production of acetaldehyde[5]:

1. Alcohol dehydrogenase (ADH). This enzyme is found in the hepatic cytosol and is the major pathway of ethanol metabolism. Multiple isoenzymes can be found in the hepatic cytosol. Catalysis of this reaction requires the conversion of NAD + to NADH.
2. Catalase. Found in the hepatocyte peroxisomes, it can metabolize ethanol into acetaldehyde through the conversion of H_2O_2 to $2H_2O$. This process catalyzes a small proportion of remaining ethanol molecules.[6]
3. P450-2E1. This microsomal enzyme also contributes to ethanol conversion to acetaldehyde, but is only significant in situations of high alcohol consumption.[7] Oxidation by this enzyme also produces highly reactive oxygen species (ROS) such as hydroxyethyl, superoxide anion, and hydroxyl radicals.[4]

The conversion of excess alcohol by ADH has 3 effects: acetaldehyde production, a decrease in the NAD+/NADH redox ratio, and mitochondrial damage that leads to a decrease in ATP production.[8] Ethanol itself can interact with membrane phospholipids, stimulate Kupffer cells, mobilize iron, decrease antioxidants, and increase oxidative stress.[9]

Excess acetaldehyde binds covalently to microtubules, resulting in the intracellular retention of normally excreted proteins and the subsequent swelling of the hepatocyte.[10] Increased acetaldehyde concentration also leads to increased production of ROS.[9] Acetaldehyde is further metabolized to acetate via acetaldehyde dehydrogenase (ALDH) generating NADH.[11] Excess NADH leads to mitochondrial oxidation that leads to further production of ROS.[11] Disulfiram, a drug used to create aversion to alcohol, blocks ALDH and causes the well-known disulfiram reaction consisting of flushing, tachycardia, nausea, thirst, chest pain, vertigo, and hypotension.

The isoenzyme ALDH2 is commonly deficient among Asians, explaining the high proportion of intolerance to alcohol in this population.[12]

THE ROLE OF KUPFFER CELLS IN ALCOHOL-INDUCED LIVER INJURY

Although the hepatocyte has classically been the center of attention of alcohol-induced liver injury, it appears that the Kupffer cell plays several key roles in the hepatotoxicity of ethanol.

In rodent models, the inactivation of Kupffer cells by gadolinium chloride almost completely prevented liver injury in rats treated with hepatotoxic levels of alcohol[13] and significantly reduced hypoxemia and the hypermetabolic rate of the hepatocyte induced by alcohol.[14] This points toward the pivotal role of the Kupffer cell in alcohol-induced hepatotoxicity by several mechanisms including direct stimulation by ethanol to produce free radicals and proinflammatory cytokines[15] and its interaction with gut-derived molecules that are altered in alcoholism.[14] Indeed, the amount of LPS, a major membrane component of gram-negative bacteria (GNB) and a major proinflammatory molecule, is significantly elevated following the ingestion of ethanol. LPS may interact with Kupffer cells to mediate inflammation,[16] and treatment with antibiotics directed toward GNB can reduce LPS levels and hence reduce Kupffer cell activation.[14] Alcoholic steatohepatitis and alcoholic liver injury are also associated with the polarization of Kupffer cells toward a proinflammatory phenotype (commonly known as M1-phenotype).[17] Transformation of Kupffer cells to another anti-inflammatory phenotype (known as M2 phenotype) promotes hepatic cell senescence, which confers resistance to alcohol toxicity.[17]

In summary, the data show that Kupffer cells appear to be necessary for ethanol to cause hepatotoxicity, and they can either be directly stimulated by ethanol to produce proinflammatory cytokines, or indirectly stimulated through an ethanol-induced increase in LPS concentrations, which in turn can activate Kupffer cells.

EXTRAHEPATIC METABOLISM OF ETHANOL

The first line of ethanol elimination is in the gastric mucosa, which is a major contributor to the protection of the liver from alcohol ingestion. A high concentration of ADH isozymes is found in the gastric mucosa, leading to significant first-pass ethanol metabolism.[18] This effect is confined to the stomach; ADH is not found in the lining cells of the small intestine.[19] Ingestion of ethanol with a meal versus just water increases first-pass metabolism (30% vs 4%),[3] confirming parental advice not to drink on an empty stomach. Both the amount and activity of gastric ADH are higher in men than women, leading to higher systemic concentrations of ethanol in women for a given amount of ingested alcohol.[18] Based on the above mechanism, total or partial gastrectomy, such as in patients undergoing sleeve gastrectomy, leads to significantly higher concentrations of ethanol.[20] Gastric ADH activity may be significantly decreased in individuals with chronically high ethanol consumption.[19] One can deduce that conditions that increase or decrease gastric emptying (eg, fasting or diabetes, respectively) may affect first-pass alcohol metabolism in the stomach. Although 90% of absorbed alcohol is eliminated by oxidation in the liver, the remaining 10% is eliminated by the lungs, skin (sweat), kidneys, and pancreas.[4]

GENETIC VARIATIONS INFLUENCING ALCOHOLIC LIVER DISEASE

Various alleles control the activity of ADH. Importantly, these alleles can have significant ethnic variations. The interest in the different genetic alleles that influence alcohol metabolism has significant clinical implications, because differences in the activity of these enzymes can influence the exposure to hepatotoxic substrates. Theoretically, an increase in the activity of ADH may lead to a significant increase in the amount of acetaldehyde, thus, increasing hepatotoxicity. Further research is needed to further elucidate a tight connection between ALD and certain alleles.

The ADH1B*3 allele, which is almost exclusive among people of African descent, has been found to confer a more rapid ethanol elimination ability, which may protect fetuses exposed to alcohol and may reduce the likelihood of ALD among adolescents who drink the same amount of alcohol.[21] Individuals with the ADH1B*3 allele also appear to have less risky alcohol use patterns, and are protected in the setting of low alcohol consumption, but they are not protected when consuming higher quantities of alcohol.[22,23]

ALDH, which metabolizes acetaldehyde to acetate, may protect the cell by reducing exposure times to acetaldehyde. The ALDH2*2 allele confers a disulfiram reaction, and it is commonly present in Asian populations.[24] Possibly because of this disulfiram-like reaction, individuals harboring this dominant allele appear to be more protected against the spectrum of ALD.[24]

ROS generated during alcohol metabolism are highly reactive, and can damage lipids, proteins, and DNA. Several enzymes that counteract these oxidative stress signals include glutathione-S-transferases (GSTs) and superoxide dismutase. Mitochondria-derived ROS are detoxified to hydrogen peroxide and water by the successive action of manganese superoxide dismutase (MnSOD). Genetic variants of GST and MnSOD have been identified, and carriers of these variants have been associated with more severe liver disease in some studies.

Kupffer cells are stimulated by various triggers (ROS, lipid peroxides, and endotoxins/lipopolysaccharides) to produce several cytokines including tumor necrosis factor alpha (TNFα), interleukins, interferons, chemokines, and certain growth factors that regulate hepatic inflammation and subsequent hepatocyte injury and death. Polymorphisms in various genes coding for cytokines in ALD have been reported in various case–control studies. These polymorphic variations of the TNF-α gene leading to variable TNF-α levels have been reported in few studies. Polymorphisms in the TNF-α gene are associated with increased TNF-α expression and progression of ALD.[25]

Patatin-like phospholipase domain-containing protein 3 (PNPLA3) is a lipase that mediates the hydrolysis of triacylglycerol molecules in adipocytes. Genetic variations have been linked to the development of ALD.[26] For example, variations in PNPLA3 rs738409 have been linked to cirrhosis; the attributable risk of this allele for progression to severe ALD is 27%.[27]

A novel splice variant of HSD17B13 that encodes the hepatic lipid droplet protein hydroxysteroid 17-beta dehydrogenase 13 (rs72613567:TA) has been associated with a 42% decreased risk of ALD.[28]

Recently, genetic variants of genes involved in the metabolism of hepatic fat (PNPLA3, TM6SF2) have been associated with nonalcoholic fatty liver disease (NAFLD).[29] These variants might act in an additive fashion in the progression of ALD.

ETHANOL AND THE HUMAN MICROBIOME

Alterations to the bacterial diversity of the human gut, also termed dysbiosis, has been implicated in the pathogenesis of various disease states such as irritable bowel syndrome[30] and colorectal tumorigenesis.[31] Ethanol consumption can have direct effects on the composition of the intestinal microbiota, which in turn can have significant implications for human health.[32,33] For example, consumption of alcohol leads to a lower abundance of *Bacteroidetes* and a higher abundance of *Proteobacteria* in the colonic mucosal microbiome, and this effect can be maintained even after a long period of sobriety.[34] These changes also correlate with differences in LPS production in a subset of patients.[34] In a murine model of alcohol ingestion, ethanol had a significant impact on the intestinal microbial composition, along with systemic increases in LPS, liver steatosis, and inflammation. These changes were prevented by the administration of *Lactobacillus rhamnosus GG* (LGG).[35] LGG administration also prevented increased gut permeability as demonstrated by decreased serum levels of tight junction proteins.[35] Tight junction proteins are the main proteins responsible for maintaining the integrity of the mucosal barrier, and their disruption can aid in LPS leakage and other long term-effects such as colorectal tumorigenesis.[36]

Several other experiments have elucidated important ethanol-related changes in the microbiome that could promote or prevent the development of ALD. *Bacteroidetes* were significantly decreased, and *Actinobacteria* and *Firmicutes* were significantly increased among mice with hepatic steatosis and inflammation induced by an alcohol-containing diet, and alcohol-induced injury was prevented by pectin (a plant-derived polysaccharide) or fecal microbiota transplantation by mice that exhibited resistance to ALD despite consuming the same amount of alcohol.[37] This change was mediated by restoring depleted populations of *Bacteroidetes*.[37] Clinically, patients with chronic alcohol use may have decreased abundance of *Bacteroidetes* in the mucosa-associated bacterial microbiome.[34] Interestingly, adverse changes in the microbiome in people appear to be long-lasting, even with prolonged abstinence from alcohol.[32] Fecal microbiota transplantation from a human with severe alcoholic hepatitis into germ-free, ethanol-fed mice conferred increased gut permeability and susceptibility to hepatotoxicity. This effect was not caused by fecal transplantation from an individual who suffered from alcoholism without alcoholic hepatitis.[38] In a randomized placebo-controlled clinical trial of 7-day in-hospital administration of *Lactobacillus subtilis* and *Streptococcus faecium* among patients admitted with alcoholic hepatitis, the treatment arm showed significant improvements in LPS, TNFα, liver enzymes, and liver function tests.[39] In a pilot open-label clinical trial of nasogastric fecal microbial transplantation (FMT) in 8 male steroid-ineligible patients with alcoholic hepatitis, FMT resulted in significant improvement in indices of liver disease and survival after almost a year of follow-up.[40] This group of 8 patients was historically matched to 18 individuals who received standard of care. These findings open the way for further translational studies that could examine the potential therapeutic role of microbiome manipulation through supplementation of targeted bacteria or whole microbiome transplantation from donors resistant to alcohol-induced liver injury to recipients with clear evidence of susceptibility to ethanol.

It is important to recognize that the intestinal milieu of microorganisms is not just limited to bacteria. Fungi, archaea, protozoa, and viruses make up a large proportion of the healthy inhabitant microflora of the intestine, but research on the effects of alcohol on these microorganisms is scarce. Chronic ethanol administration in mice led to significantly increased relative abundance of fungi and systemic concentrations of β-D-glucan,[41] an important constituent of the fungal cell wall and a surrogate for the diagnosis of invasive fungal infections.[42] More specifically, proportions of *Humicola* species, *Fusarium*, and *Aspergillus* increased, while proportions of *Candida* species (especially *Candida parapsilosis*) decreased after ethanol consumption.[41] These observations on fungi are clinically important; in one of the largest hallmark clinical trials of early versus late liver transplantation among patients suffering from severe acute alcoholic hepatitis by Mathurin and colleagues,[43] 5 out of the 6 deaths after transplantation were related to systemic *Aspergillus* infection. It appears that intestinal fungal decolonization or pre-emptive antifungal therapy of early acute alcoholic hepatitis patients who are candidates for transplantation could be in important intervention. Further research in the field is required.

Intestinal bacteria and fungi have both the ability to produce ethanol and to metabolize ethanol to its by-products such as acetaldehyde and acetate, mostly through oxidation.[44,45] Administration of antibiotics reduces microbial production of alcohol as measured by circulating ethanol and acetaldehyde levels in a rodent model of small intestinal bacterial overgrowth (SIBO).[45] In the same model, rats with higher intestinal bacterial numbers had a blunted increase in systemic circulation of ethanol and its by-products compared with controls, emphasizing that the net effect of bacterial production versus metabolism of ethanol in an SIBO model leads to overall decreases in the concentrations of ethanol or ethanol by-products.

Whether the presence of SIBO or higher abundance of specific microorganisms in the human intestine could translate into a blunted response to ethanol ingestion has not been thoroughly investigated. This may be clinically relevant, because the prevalence of SIBO among individuals with cirrhosis may be around 30%.[46] In addition, intestinal transit is reduced among patients with cirrhosis who drink alcohol,[47,48] which may variably influence bacterial overgrowth. The implication of such findings could be that consumption of alcohol among individuals who suffer from cirrhosis might not be as easily detectable, and that detection of serum alcohol in these individuals might mean an actually higher consumption than the what one would conclude based solely on alcohol detection methods.

IS MODERATE CONSUMPTION OF ETHANOL SAFE OR PROTECTIVE?

Moderate consumption of ethanol is defined as up to 1 standard drink per day for women and up to 2 standard drinks per day for men. Moderate consumption of ethanol is considered safe from a public health standpoint, but some data show that moderate consumption might still lead to alterations in the gut microbiome of both rats and people that could potentially be pathogenic.[49] A robust meta-analysis on the global burden of ALD has pinpointed that even 1 standard drink per day might be harmful, specifically raising the risk of all-cause mortality and cancer-related mortality.[1] On the other hand, moderate alcohol consumption reduced endotoxemia among individuals with fatty liver in large population-based studies, pointing to the protective effect of alcohol for the development of NAFLD or nonalcoholic steatohepatitis in these individuals.[50]

A recent analysis of the effects of moderate alcohol consumption showed significant shifts in the overall diversity of the gut microbial communities and a dramatic change in the relative abundance of particular microbes such as the lactobacilli. *Lactobacillus* species are significantly suppressed following chronic ingestion of ethanol, and this effect is sustained even after stopping ethanol consumption.[51]

Genetic variations that cause decreased ALDH activity may lead to higher peaks of acetaldehyde compared with normal controls even with mild-to-moderate alcohol consumption.[52] It is important to recognize these variations and develop specific guidelines that define a healthy amount of alcohol consumption in these individuals.

OTHER MECHANISMS OF ETHANOL-INDUCED LIVER DISEASE

From an epidemiologic standpoint, it is clear that the amount and duration of alcohol exposure leads to significant hepatotoxicity.[53] However, the exact mechanisms by which alcohol exerts its effects remain under investigation. A breakthrough in alcohol-induced liver injury involved the development of a murine model of ALD by Tsukamoto and French.[54,55] Rodent models of alcohol liver injury have uncovered significant key mediators of alcohol-induced liver injury.

INFLUENCE OF THE ENVIRONMENT

Environmental pollutants have a tangible risk for the progression of several liver diseases, including alcohol related liver disease. These environmental factors may be difficult to identify, and are not usually included in studies that examine the pathogenesis of ALD.[56] For example, arsenic can be naturally found in the environment, and people are routinely exposed to it through food, water, air, and soil.[57] A common constituent of pesticides, chemotherapies and various household products, arsenic can reach significant levels in certain individuals. The presence of inorganic arsenic may potentiate the effect of ethanol in the development of ALD.[58] In another example, environmental exposure to benzo[a]pyrene (B[a]P) has also been shown to induce progression to steatohepatitis among alcohol-treated hepatocytes and in a zebrafish model.[59] Further exploration of environmental pollutants and their effects on ALD is beyond the scope of this article and can be reviewed elsewhere.[56]

REFERENCES

1. GBD 2016 Alcohol Collaborators. Alcohol use and burden for 195 countries and territories, 1990-2016: a systematic analysis for the global burden of disease study. Lancet 2018;392(10152):1015–35.
2. Cortot A, Jobin G, Ducrot F, et al. Gastric emptying and gastrointestinal absorption of alcohol ingested with a meal. Dig Dis Sci 1986;31(4):343–8.
3. Levitt MD, Li R, DeMaster EG, et al. Use of measurements of ethanol absorption from stomach and intestine to assess human ethanol metabolism. Am J Physiol 1997;273(4 Pt 1):G951–7.
4. Sanyal AJ, Boyer T, Terrault N, et al. Zakim and Boyer's hepatology: a textbook of liver disease. USA: Elsevier; 2017.
5. Edenberg HJ. The genetics of alcohol metabolism: role of alcohol dehydrogenase and aldehyde dehydrogenase variants. Alcohol Res Health 2007;30(1): 5–13.
6. Handler JA, Thurman RG. Catalase-dependent ethanol oxidation in perfused rat liver. Requirement for fatty-acid-stimulated H_2O_2 production by peroxisomes. Eur J Biochem 1988;176(2):477–84.
7. Lieber CS, DeCarli LM. Ethanol oxidation by hepatic microsomes: adaptive increase after ethanol feeding. Science 1968;162(3856):917–8.
8. Cederbaum AI, Lu Y, Wu D. Role of oxidative stress in alcohol-induced liver injury. Arch Toxicol 2009;83(6):519–48.
9. Wu D, Cederbaum AI. Oxidative stress and alcoholic liver disease. Semin Liver Dis 2009;29(2):141–54.
10. Lieber CS. Metabolic effects of acetaldehyde. Biochem Soc Trans 1988;16(3): 241–7.
11. Cederbaum AI. Alcohol metabolism. Clin Liver Dis 2012;16(4):667–85.

12. Bosron WF, Ehrig T, Li TK. Genetic factors in alcohol metabolism and alcoholism. Semin Liver Dis 1993;13(2):126–35.
13. Adachi Y, Bradford BU, Gao W, et al. Inactivation of Kupffer cells prevents early alcohol-induced liver injury. Hepatology 1994;20(2):453–60.
14. Adachi Y, Moore LE, Bradford BU, et al. Antibiotics prevent liver injury in rats following long-term exposure to ethanol. Gastroenterology 1995;108(1):218–24.
15. Wheeler MD, Kono H, Yin M, et al. The role of Kupffer cell oxidant production in early ethanol-induced liver disease. Free Radic Biol Med 2001;31(12):1544–9.
16. Nanji AA, Khettry U, Sadrzadeh SM, et al. Severity of liver injury in experimental alcoholic liver disease. Correlation with plasma endotoxin, prostaglandin E2, leukotriene B4, and thromboxane B2. Am J Pathol 1993;142(2):367–73.
17. Wan J, Benkdane M, Alons E, et al. M2 Kupffer cells promote hepatocyte senescence: an IL-6-dependent protective mechanism against alcoholic liver disease. Am J Pathol 2014;184(6):1763–72.
18. Frezza M, di Padova C, Pozzato G, et al. High blood alcohol levels in women. The role of decreased gastric alcohol dehydrogenase activity and first-pass metabolism. N Engl J Med 1990;322(2):95–9.
19. Lieber CS, Gentry RT, Baraona E. First pass metabolism of ethanol. Alcohol Alcohol Suppl 1994;2:163–9.
20. Maluenda F, Csendes A, De Aretxabala X, et al. Alcohol absorption modification after a laparoscopic sleeve gastrectomy due to obesity. Obes Surg 2010;20(6):744–8.
21. Dodge NC, Jacobson JL, Jacobson SW. Protective effects of the alcohol dehydrogenase-ADH1B*3 allele on attention and behavior problems in adolescents exposed to alcohol during pregnancy. Neurotoxicol Teratol 2014;41:43–50.
22. Zaso MJ, Desalu JM, Kim J, et al. Interaction between the ADH1B*3 allele and drinking motives on alcohol use among Black college students. Am J Drug Alcohol Abuse 2018;44(3):329–38.
23. Desalu JM, Zaso MJ, Kim J, et al. Interaction between ADH1B*3 and alcohol-facilitating social environments in alcohol behaviors among college students of African descent. Am J Addict 2017;26(4):349–56.
24. Borras E, Coutelle C, Rosell A, et al. Genetic polymorphism of alcohol dehydrogenase in Europeans: the ADH2*2 allele decreases the risk for alcoholism and is associated with ADH3*1. Hepatology 2000;31(4):984–9.
25. Marcos M, Gomez-Munuera M, Pastor I, et al. Tumor necrosis factor polymorphisms and alcoholic liver disease: a HuGE review and meta-analysis. Am J Epidemiol 2009;170(8):948–56.
26. Kolla BP, Schneekloth TD, Biernacka J, et al. PNPLA3 association with alcoholic liver disease in a cohort of heavy drinkers. Alcohol Alcohol 2018;53(4):357–60.
27. Stickel F, Buch S, Lau K, et al. Genetic variation in the PNPLA3 gene is associated with alcoholic liver injury in Caucasians. Hepatology 2011;53(1):86–95.
28. Abul-Husn NS, Cheng X, Li AH, et al. A protein-truncating HSD17B13 variant and protection from chronic liver disease. N Engl J Med 2018;378(12):1096–106.
29. Sliz E, Sebert S, Wurtz P, et al. NAFLD risk alleles in PNPLA3, TM6SF2, GCKR and LYPLAL1 show divergent metabolic effects. Hum Mol Genet 2018;27(12):2214–23.
30. Collins SM. A role for the gut microbiota in IBS. Nat Rev Gastroenterol Hepatol 2014;11(8):497–505.
31. Sobhani I, Amiot A, Le Baleur Y, et al. Microbial dysbiosis and colon carcinogenesis: could colon cancer be considered a bacteria-related disease? Therap Adv Gastroenterol 2013;6(3):215–29.

32. Woodhouse CA, Patel VC, Singanayagam A, et al. Review article: the gut micro-biome as a therapeutic target in the pathogenesis and treatment of chronic liver disease. Aliment Pharmacol Ther 2018;47(2):192–202.

33. Engen PA, Green SJ, Voigt RM, et al. The gastrointestinal microbiome: alcohol effects on the composition of intestinal microbiota. Alcohol Res 2015;37(2):223–36.

34. Mutlu EA, Gillevet PM, Rangwala H, et al. Colonic microbiome is altered in alcoholism. Am J Physiol Gastrointest Liver Physiol 2012;302(9):G966–78.

35. Bull-Otterson L, Feng W, Kirpich I, et al. Metagenomic analyses of alcohol induced pathogenic alterations in the intestinal microbiome and the effect of *Lactobacillus rhamnosus* GG treatment. PLoS One 2013;8(1):e53028.

36. Kourkoumpetis Themistoklis RK, Chen L, Ravishankar M, et al. Differential expression of tight junctions and cell polarity genes in human colon cancer. Explor Res Hypothesis Med 2018;3(1):14–9.

37. Ferrere G, Wrzosek L, Cailleux F, et al. Fecal microbiota manipulation prevents dysbiosis and alcohol-induced liver injury in mice. J Hepatol 2017;66(4):806–15.

38. Llopis M, Cassard AM, Wrzosek L, et al. Intestinal microbiota contributes to individual susceptibility to alcoholic liver disease. Gut 2016;65(5):830–9.

39. Han SH, Suk KT, Kim DJ, et al. Effects of probiotics (cultured *Lactobacillus subtilis/Streptococcus faecium*) in the treatment of alcoholic hepatitis: randomized-controlled multicenter study. Eur J Gastroenterol Hepatol 2015;27(11):1300–6.

40. Philips CA, Pande A, Shasthry SM, et al. Healthy donor fecal microbiota transplantation in steroid-ineligible severe alcoholic hepatitis: a pilot study. Clin Gastroenterol Hepatol 2017;15(4):600–2.

41. Yang AM, Inamine T, Hochrath K, et al. Intestinal fungi contribute to development of alcoholic liver disease. J Clin Invest 2017;127(7):2829–41.

42. Kourkoumpetis TK, Fuchs BB, Coleman JJ, et al. Polymerase chain reaction-based assays for the diagnosis of invasive fungal infections. Clin Infect Dis 2012;54(9):1322–31.

43. Mathurin P, Moreno C, Samuel D, et al. Early liver transplantation for severe alcoholic hepatitis. N Engl J Med 2011;365(19):1790–800.

44. Krebs HA, Perkins JR. The physiological role of liver alcohol dehydrogenase. Biochem J 1970;118(4):635–44.

45. Baraona E, Julkunen R, Tannenbaum L, et al. Role of intestinal bacterial overgrowth in ethanol production and metabolism in rats. Gastroenterology 1986; 90(1):103–10.

46. Casafont Morencos F, de las Heras Castano G, Martin Ramos L, et al. Small bowel bacterial overgrowth in patients with alcoholic cirrhosis. Dig Dis Sci 1996;41(3):552–6.

47. Sadik R, Abrahamsson H, Bjornsson E, et al. Etiology of portal hypertension may influence gastrointestinal transit. Scand J Gastroenterol 2003;38(10):1039–44.

48. Usami M, Miyoshi M, Yamashita H. Gut microbiota and host metabolism in liver cirrhosis. World J Gastroenterol 2015;21(41):11597–608.

49. Kosnicki KL, Penprase JC, Cintora P, et al. Effects of moderate, voluntary ethanol consumption on the rat and human gut microbiome. Addict Biol 2018. [Epub ahead of print].

50. Wong VW, Wong GL, Chan HY, et al. Bacterial endotoxin and non-alcoholic fatty liver disease in the general population: a prospective cohort study. Aliment Pharmacol Ther 2015;42(6):731–40.

51. Yan AW, Fouts DE, Brandl J, et al. Enteric dysbiosis associated with a mouse model of alcoholic liver disease. Hepatology 2011;53(1):96–105.

52. Enomoto N, Takase S, Yasuhara M, et al. Acetaldehyde metabolism in different aldehyde dehydrogenase-2 genotypes. Alcohol Clin Exp Res 1991;15(1):141–4.
53. Mann RE, Smart RG, Govoni R. The epidemiology of alcoholic liver disease. Alcohol Res Health 2003;27(3):209–19.
54. Tsukamoto H, Reidelberger RD, French SW, et al. Long-term cannulation model for blood sampling and intragastric infusion in the rat. Am J Physiol 1984;247(3 Pt 2):R595–9.
55. French SW, Miyamoto K, Tsukamoto H. Ethanol-induced hepatic fibrosis in the rat: role of the amount of dietary fat. Alcohol Clin Exp Res 1986;10(6 Suppl):13S–9S.
56. Arciello M, Gori M, Maggio R, et al. Environmental pollution: a tangible risk for NAFLD pathogenesis. Int J Mol Sci 2013;14(11):22052–66.
57. Hughes MF, Beck BD, Chen Y, et al. Arsenic exposure and toxicology: a historical perspective. Toxicol Sci 2011;123(2):305–32.
58. Bambino K, Zhang C, Austin C, et al. Inorganic arsenic causes fatty liver and interacts with ethanol to cause alcoholic liver disease in zebrafish. Dis Model Mech 2018;11(2) [pii:dmm031575].
59. Bucher S, Tete A, Podechard N, et al. Co-exposure to benzo[a]pyrene and ethanol induces a pathological progression of liver steatosis in vitro and in vivo. Sci Rep 2018;8(1):5963.

Acute Alcoholic Hepatitis

Gene Y. Im, MD

KEYWORDS

- Alcoholic hepatitis • Alcohol use disorder • Discriminant function • Lille score
- Corticosteroids • Pentoxifylline • *N*-acetylcysteine • Hepatorenal syndrome

KEY POINTS

- Acute alcoholic hepatitis is a serious form of liver inflammation caused by prolonged heavy alcohol consumption that carries a significant mortality risk.
- In its early or milder presentations, alcoholic hepatitis is difficult to detect, requiring nonjudgmental provider engagement with a potential role for transient elastography.
- Scoring systems like the Maddrey Discriminant Function, Model for End-stage Liver Disease, and Lille model should be used to assess prognosis and guide treatment.
- Prednisolone 40 mg/d given orally or its equivalent is recommended for patients with severe alcoholic hepatitis (discriminant function of ≥32) in the absence of contraindications.

INTRODUCTION

Alcoholic hepatitis (AH) is a unique type of alcohol-associated liver disease (ALD) characterized by acute liver inflammation caused by prolonged heavy alcohol use. The short-term prognosis of acute AH depends on liver recovery, and ranges widely from rapid improvement with supportive care to grim multiorgan failure despite treatment. Recent advances in the treatment of AH have reinforced corticosteroids as the cornerstone of treatment, used for more than 4 decades, to enhance short-term survival.

ALD is now the leading liver disease indication for liver transplantation in the United States. Recent trends of increasing alcohol use disorder (AUD) in the United States and effective therapies for hepatitis C virus have likely contributed to ALD's emergence as the leading indication for liver transplantation in the United States.

EVENTS PRECEDING THE ONSET OF ALCOHOLIC HEPATITIS

AH is an acute, inflammatory syndrome of jaundice and liver injury occurring in a subset of patients, typically after decades of heavy alcohol use (mean intake of 100 g [8–10 drinks] per day).[1–3] Before the onset of jaundice, patients with heavy

Disclosure Statement: The author has nothing to disclose.
Division of Liver Diseases, Icahn School of Medicine at Mount Sinai, Recanati-Miller Transplantation Institute, One Gustave Levy Place, Box 1104, New York, NY 10029, USA
E-mail address: gene.im@mountsinai.org

Clin Liver Dis 23 (2019) 81–98
https://doi.org/10.1016/j.cld.2018.09.005
1089-3261/19/© 2018 Elsevier Inc. All rights reserved.

alcohol use of greater than 60 g/d develop alcohol-associated fatty liver, which is typically asymptomatic.[4] Subtle stigmata of this condition include hepatic steatosis with or without hepatomegaly and mild liver enzymes elevations, particularly aspartate aminotransferase and gamma glutamyltransferase. The evolution from heavy drinking to fatty liver to alcoholic steatohepatitis (the distinct histopathologic correlate of AH) is rarely linear, but rather has progression and regression depending on several factors, including periods of reduction or abstinence from alcohol.[5] This plasticity requires providers to have a high index of suspicion for excessive alcohol use in patients with mild liver injury and nonspecific signs and symptoms. The presence of concomitant conditions like obesity (possibly with nonalcoholic steatohepatitis), viral hepatitis, and human immunodeficiency virus infection may also influence the progression and severity of superimposed AH. There are many other factors (genetic, environmental) that influence the risk of alcohol-associated liver injury that are beyond the scope of this review.

DIAGNOSIS

The excessive use of alcohol and AH are inextricably linked. Because there are no diagnostic tests for AH, eliciting an accurate history of alcohol use from a patient is paramount to its diagnosis. This process may be challenging for several reasons. First, a patient may not be forthright in providing a factual drinking history. Second, a provider may not be familiar or comfortable with appropriate interview techniques. The provider should ask about current and past alcohol consumption in a nonjudgmental way to obtain an accurate response, because patterns of alcohol use can change over time.[6] Patients with AH often have been abstinent from alcohol for several weeks before their presentation.[1] Thus, it is important to obtain histories over discrete time periods, particularly related to recent life stressors causing increased consumption.[7] This approach is particularly useful in assessing the impact of alcohol in more equivocal situations of liver injury where concomitant conditions such as nonalcoholic fatty liver disease, drug-induced liver injury, or viral hepatitis may be confounding. Third, even agreeing on what constitutes a standard drink can be confusing and complicated by the use of jargon such as jigger, forty, handle, quart, and fifth, and provider unfamiliarity.[8-10]

The often surreptitious nature of excessive drinking with or without AUD, low rates of engagement with providers, and the protean presentation of AH makes early detection difficult. In a nationally representative survey of 648 primary care providers in the United States, 94% failed to identify AUD as 1 of their 5 possible diagnoses in a hypothetical vignette, with only 1 in 5 providers considering themselves very prepared to identify AUD.[11] This missed opportunity at the medical front-line contributes to presentation at later stages of disease with higher financial and societal costs. For instance, more than 50% of patients with symptomatic AH present with advanced liver disease and nearly all with severe AH already have cirrhosis.[5,12]

The presentation of acute AH is varied, ranging from asymptomatic to overt liver failure. Acute AH is a clinical syndrome characterized by jaundice (serum bilirubin >3 mg/dL) and elevated aspartate aminotransferase and ALT (aspartate aminotransferase to ALT ratio >1.5 but <400 IU/mL), with a history of heavy alcohol use. In cases of milder liver enzyme elevation with an ambiguous alcohol history, the validated ALD/NAFLD (nonalcoholic fatty liver disease) Index can assist in differentiating between AH and nonalcoholic steatohepatitis.[13] Although the minimum amount of alcohol use to cause AH is unknown, common parameters are more than 3 drinks per day for women and more than 4 drinks per day for men for more than

6 months recently (usually >5 years lifetime) with fewer than 60 days of abstinence before the onset of jaundice.[4] Sarcopenia, malaise, tender hepatomegaly, and symptoms of hepatic decompensation are common, but not specific to AH. Ultrasound examination (to avoid the use of nephrotoxic intravenous contrast agents) to exclude biliary obstruction, and serologic testing for viral hepatitis, autoimmune liver diseases, and Wilson disease should be performed.

Fitting an individual patient into the myriad features constituting the syndrome of AH can be challenging, with inaccuracy of a purely clinical diagnosis ranging from 4% to 46%.[14–19] Thus, a liver biopsy can be useful to confirm the diagnosis, rule out the other diagnoses found in 10% to 20% of cases, and for prognostication.[20,21] However, performing routine liver biopsy for AH has its challenges in clinical practice. Because most patients with severe AH have cirrhosis, many have portal hypertension, either chronically or as a consequence of AH. Therefore, many of these patients have coagulation derangements (especially those with a low fibrinogen concentration and/or platelets of <50,000) with an increased risk of bleeding. In addition, liver biopsy cannot distinguish between alcoholic steatohepatitis and nonalcoholic steatohepatitis.[22] Most liver programs in the United States have adopted a transjugular biopsy route for AH diagnosis, but this procedure is not performed routinely given its associated risks and cost. In contrast, liver biopsy is common practice in Europe, where it is often performed by hepatologists.[1]

A review of 11 randomized, controlled trials of biopsy-proven AH demonstrated that 1409 of 1668 biopsies (84.5%) showed histologic evidence of AH and that the addition of a total bilirubin of greater than 80 µmol/L (>4.7 mg/dL) increased the accuracy of AH diagnosis to 96%.[19] In a more recent retrospective study of patients with a clinical presentation suggestive of AH where liver biopsy was the gold standard for diagnosing AH, the combination of an elevated leukocyte count and nodular liver surface on imaging, in the absence of active infection, retrospectively identified patients with a high likelihood of histologic AH.[23]

A recent consensus statement from members of the National Institute on Alcohol Abuse and Alcoholism–funded Alcoholic Hepatitis Consortia regarding the clinical diagnosis AH, and when biopsy confirmation of alcoholic steatohepatitis was optimal to improve consistency between studies and in clinical trials was published in 2017 (**Box 1**). It categorizes patients with putative AH into 3 groups: those with definitive biopsy-proven AH, those with probable AH, and those with possible AH requiring biopsy confirmation of histologic features of alcoholic steatohepatitis (eg, to enroll in a clinical trial). These definitions can also provide diagnostic guidance for clinical decision making, particularly in challenging cases. The role of liver biopsy is, therefore, to resolve cases of diagnostic uncertainty and develop consistency for AH clinical trials.

Acute-on-Chronic Liver Failure

Another complicating factor in the diagnosis of AH is the distinction between AH and acute-on-chronic liver failure (ACLF). ACLF is a relatively new concept in hepatology, encompassing a subset of patients with cirrhosis with rapidly progressive decompensation, multiorgan failure, and high short-term mortality.[24] Although the etiologies of ACLF differ worldwide, recent alcohol use is a common precipitating factor in the pathogenesis of ACLF. Because nearly all patients with severe AH are already cirrhotic and often present with multiorgan dysfunction, it is likely that a significant proportion of ACLF is superimposed in severe AH.[25] Given the diagnostic difficulties described elsewhere in this article, alcohol-associated ACLF is likely underreported and possibly constitutes a significant proportion of the ACLF of unknown origin, regardless of

---

Box 1
Consensus definitions for the diagnosis of alcoholic hepatitis

Clinical diagnosis of AH (minimum criteria)
- Onset of jaundice within prior 8 weeks
- Ongoing consumption of greater than 40 (female) or 60 (males) g alcohol/d for 6 or more months, with less than 60 days of abstinence before the onset of jaundice
- AST greater than 50, AST/ALT greater than 1.5, and both values less than 400 IU/L
- Serum bilirubin (total) greater than 3.0 mg/dL

Definite AH: Clinically diagnosed and biopsy proven. In the future, imaging techniques and biomarkers may replace liver biopsy for definite diagnosis of AH.

Probable AH: Clinically diagnosed AH without confounding factors (see below).
- In patients with heavy alcohol use and typical liver tests; and negative markers for immune (ANA <1:160 or ASMA <1:80 dilutions) and metabolic liver disease; and absence of sepsis, shock, cocaine use, or recent use of a drug with DILI potential within 30 days.
- Patients with positive tests for HBV, HCV, or NASH do not commonly present in a fashion mimicking AH.

Possible AH: Clinically diagnosed but with potential confounding factors, including possible ischemic hepatitis (eg, severe upper gastrointestinal bleed, hypotension, or cocaine use within 7 days); possible DILI; uncertain alcohol use assessment (eg, patient denies excessive alcohol use); and atypical laboratory tests (eg, AST of <50 IU/mL or >400 IU/mL, AST/ALT ratio of <1.5), ANA greater than 1:160 or SMA greater than 1:80. *Biopsy needed for confirmation of AH.*

Abbreviations: AH, alcoholic hepatitis; ALT, alanine aminotransferase; ANA, anti-nuclear antibody; ASMA, anti–smooth antibody; AST, aspartate aminotransferase; DILI, drug-induced liver injury; HBV, hepatitis B virus; HCV, hepatitis C virus; NASH, nonalcoholic steatohepatitis.

---

geography.[26] Whether conventional AH-specific therapies are effective in patients with alcohol-associated ACLF is currently unknown.

Alcoholic Hepatitis Detection Strategies

Although there are multiple validated questionnaire and biomarker tests for AUD and recent heavy drinking, the field of liver-specific early detection strategies for AH and other forms of ALD is in its infancy. Indirect testing for AH through the detection of liver fibrosis in the appropriate clinical context is a promising strategy. Elastography by ultrasound examination or MRI can assess liver stiffness as a surrogate for liver fibrosis and is becoming more widely available. Because inflammation also increases liver stiffness, testing in the acute phase of AH can lead to falsely elevated measurements. Recognition that restoration of liver elasticity occurs with abstinence in patients with AH is important for test interpretation.[27] Transient elastography and serum liver fibrosis markers like Enhanced Liver Fibrosis test and FibroTest have recently been assessed as noninvasive screening methods for early or mild ALD. Thiele and colleagues[28] prospectively evaluated 199 patients with AUD without known liver disease with transient elastography and same-day liver biopsies and demonstrated that transient elastography accurately diagnosed significant fibrosis in ALD (area under the curve of ≥ 0.92) with a high negative predictive value. Of note, despite enrolling asymptomatic patients with normal or only slightly abnormal liver blood tests, nearly one-half (42%) had significant fibrosis (Ishak score of ≥ 3, Metavir F of ≥ 2). The proposed threshold of 9.6 kPa (Ishak score of ≥ 3, Metavir F of ≥ 2) was similar to a recent meta-analysis of individual patient data proposing 9.0 kPa as the threshold for a Metavir F of 2 or greater. The Enhanced Liver Fibrosis test and FibroTest performed similarly well in detecting fibrosis (area under the curve of 0.90) using thresholds of 10.5 and 0.58, respectively; however, the addition of these serum markers to transient elastography did not improve accuracy.[29] Although showing promise as inexpensive, noninvasive screening tools for AH and ALD, these results require further study and validation outside of Europe.

Mallory-Denk bodies are a classic, but not pathognomonic, histologic feature of alcohol-associated steatohepatitis. They are cytoplasmic inclusions representing rearrangements of the cell cytoskeleton from ethanol injury, of which the main constituent is cytokeratin-18. After apoptosis and necrosis, cytokeratin-18 fragments can be released into the plasma by hepatocytes, and may thus reflect hepatocyte cell death. Recently, plasma levels of circulating cytokeratin-18 fragments (M65 and M30) were measured in patients with biopsy-proven AH, demonstrating good accuracy (area under the curve of 0.84).[30] This AH-specific serum biomarker requires further study, but has future potential as a diagnostic tool that may further obviate the need for liver biopsy.

ASSESSING PROGNOSIS IN ALCOHOLIC HEPATITIS

There are several validated scoring systems that can be used to assess the severity and short-term prognosis of AH (**Table 1**). There are many overlapping variables between the laboratory-based scores that are easily and quickly obtained. Providers should use smartphone or online calculators to obtain these scores to help guide clinical decision making. Although these scoring systems perform similarly well in predicting AH outcome, there are advantages and disadvantages to each that are discussed.[31,32]

Discriminant Function

The discriminant function (DF) was derived from a prospective, double-blind, placebo-controlled trial of prednisolone for AH, and later modified to account for variations in prothrombin time (PT) measurement.[33] Patients with a DF of greater than or equal to 32 had a 1-month mortality of 30% to 50% with a 30-day survival benefit if given prednisolone. The DF is highly sensitive to identifying patients with AH at risk of early mortality and is time-tested as the near-universal criterion for clinical trials in AH.

Table 1
Characteristics of lab-based scoring systems in alcoholic hepatitis

	Bili	PT/ INR	Cr/ BUN	Age	Alb	WBC	Stratification	Clinical Use
MDF	+	+	—	—	—	—	Severe: ≥32	Start CS
MELD	+	+	+	—	—	—	Severe: ≥21, but a continuous scale	Prognosis only
ABIC	+	+	+	+	—	—	High mortality risk: >9 Intermediate: 6.71–9.00 Low: <6.71	Prognosis only
GAHS	+	+	+	+	—	+	Poor prognosis: ≥9	Start CS if ≥9 and MDF ≥32
Lille	+	+	+	+	+	—	≥0.45: Nonresponse <0.45: Response	Day 7 cessation or continuation of CS

Abbreviations: ABIC, age, serum bilirubin, INR, and serum creatinine; Alb, albumin; Bili, total bilirubin; Cr/BUN, creatinine/blood urea nitrogen; CS, corticosteroids; GAHS, Glasgow Alcoholic Hepatitis Score; MDF, Maddrey discriminant function; MELD, Model for End-stage Liver Disease; PT/INR, prothrombin time/international normalized ratio; WBC, white blood cell count.

However, its specificity is suboptimal because many patients with a DF of greater than or equal to 32 survive even without AH-specific treatment. In contrast, a DF of less than 32 accurately identifies those with mild to moderate AH with a low risk of mortality with supportive care. The DF is also limited as a static, dichotomous variable calculated at the time of presentation. Additionally, the DF uses PT and control PT rather than the international normalized ratio. In the United States, the control PT is not commonly reported and usually requires a managing provider to contact the laboratory to confirm the correct value (usually the mean of the reference range). Because control PT values can differ by laboratory and change over time based on the reagents used and methodology, attention should be paid to this issue, especially in retrospective clinical research.[34,35] Although the DF calculation can be a source of confusion in clinical use, the model is still widely used in both clinical practice and research.

Lille Model

The Lille model codifies the clinical observation that an early change in bilirubin levels after starting corticosteroids was associated with improved prognosis.[36] The addition of this dynamic variable of comparing bilirubin levels at days 0 and 7 is a key feature of this validated model. The Lille model differs from other prediction models in that it was designed to influence clinical decision making by augmenting the DF to assess the likelihood of response to corticosteroids in a well-characterized, biopsy-proven cohort of patients with AH with a DF of greater than or equal to 32.[37] The model helps to answer the question of whether a patient with severe AH should continue receiving corticosteroids after 7 days as a responder to medical therapy. A Lille score of less than or equal to 0.25 predicts a good response to corticosteroids and a 25% mortality rate at 6 months. In contrast, a Lille score of greater than or equal to 0.45 predicts a poor response (supporting cessation of therapy) and a 75% mortality rate. A subsequent pooled metaanalysis of individual data confirmed the 28-day survival benefit of corticosteroids according to a tripartite classification of the Lille score: complete responders (score <0.16; <35th percentile), partial responders (score 0.16–0.56; 35th-70th percentile), and null responders (score >0.56; >70th percentile).[38] The corresponding 28-day mortality rates were 9%, 21%, and 47%, respectively. Corticosteroids improved survival in complete and partial responders, but not in null responders (Lille >0.56), a higher threshold that increases eligibility to continue corticosteroids. Recently, a study demonstrated that calculating the Lille score after 4 days had similar accuracy in determining response, potentially decreasing unnecessary exposure to corticosteroids even further.[39]

Model for End-Stage Liver Disease

As in other areas of hepatology, the Model for End-stage Liver Disease (MELD) score has also been applied to and validated in AH. The MELD score accurately predicts outcome in AH and has the benefit of capturing renal function, which has been independently associated with outcomes in severe AH.[40] The MELD score may give a falsely poor prognosis in cases where liver function is improving in the setting of persistent poor renal function. The MELD score is also valued as a commonly used continuous model that can be measured at different time points to assess prognosis. However, the MELD score threshold defining poor prognosis at which corticosteroids or other medical therapies are useful has not been established. A MELD score of greater than 20 has been proposed by consensus opinion, particularly with a minimum total bilirubin of 5 mg/dL and an increasing MELD score of at least 2 in the first week.[41,42] Additionally, its use has been studied and verified in ACLF.[24,43]

Glasgow Alcoholic Hepatitis Score

The Glasgow Alcoholic Hepatitis Score (GAHS) was derived and validated in a study population that did not receive corticosteroids or pentoxifylline.[44] The score considers age and white blood cell count in addition to shared variables with the other models. Although the GAHS has been shown to have greater accuracy and specificity compared with the DF or the MELD score, it is less sensitive in predicting 1- and 3-month mortality. Given the high risk of short-term mortality, an AH model would preferably have a high sensitivity to identifying all patients with AH at risk. The GAHS most useful role may be as an adjunct to the DF. A GAHS of 9 or greater (plus a DF of >32) identified patients benefiting from corticosteroids, compared with a GAHS of less than 9, where no benefit of corticosteroids was found.[45] Although not validated outside the UK, it may decrease the number of patients needed to treat with corticosteroids to achieve a favorable response.

Age, Serum Bilirubin, International Normalized Ratio, and Serum Creatinine Model

The age, serum bilirubin, international normalized ratio, and serum creatinine (ABIC) model is a newer prediction model, derived and validated in a Spanish biopsy-proven AH cohort, that stratifies patients into low, intermediate, and high risk of mortality at 90 days and 1 year.[46] Because the ABIC model was developed in a cohort treated with corticosteroids, it is likely limited as a tool to identify patients best suited to treatment with corticosteroids. As with the MELD score, it incorporates renal function, but lacks a threshold informing when corticosteroids should be started.

Joint-Effect Combinative Models

A recent study evaluated various combinations of the dynamic Lille model with static models for outcome prediction in AH.[47] These joint-effect combinative models originated in a corticosteroid-treated European cohort and were validated in a similar multinational cohort. Although all combinations performed well, the MELD plus Lille combination was better at predicting survival at 2 and 6 months than the DF plus Lille or ABIC plus Lille combinations and single models, with an area under the curve of 0.77. These combinative models, particularly MELD plus Lille, provide a continuum of mortality risk from 0% to 100% instead of a tiered prognosis, allowing for a more nuanced and precise prediction of outcome, particularly for intermediate risk. Thus, the MELD plus Lille joint-effect model has significant value for patient management and the design of future clinical trials. It can also be easily calculated online at www.lillemodel.com.

Alcoholic Hepatitis Histologic Score

The Alcoholic Hepatitis Histologic Score (AHHS) was developed and refined in a multinational effort as the first histologic AH prediction model.[21] The AHHS is semiquantitative with histologic variables previously correlated with AH prognosis. Of note, mild or absent neutrophil infiltration confers points toward a higher risk of mortality compared with severe neutrophil infiltration. This factor may seem contrary to a higher serum white blood cell count conferring higher risk in the GAHS and Lille model, with a feature of systemic inflammatory response syndrome (SIRS) likely playing an unascertained role.[48] The AHHS requires an early liver biopsy obtained within 48 hours of admission to be scored correctly, which limits its practical applicability given patient safety, availability of transjugular biopsy, and cost concerns. Whereas the ABIC model and AHHS are organizationally similar with 3 tiers of risk, caution is advised in directly comparing these or other models. For example, the low-, intermediate-, and high-risk mortality rates for the ABIC model and AHHS vary widely (3% vs 0%, 19% vs 30%, and 51% vs 75%, respectively). Prospective, real-world evaluation of the AHHS is needed.

Gene-Signature Plus Model-for End-Stage Liver Disease Score

In a proof-of-principle study to incorporate gene expression profiles in alcoholic steatohepatitis liver tissue with clinical variables, Trépo and colleagues[49] derived the gene-signature plus MELD (gs-MELD) scoring system. By combining the expression patterns of 123 genes with the MELD score, this study distinguished patients with poor and good 90-day survival with good accuracy (area under the curve of 0.86) and outperformed other laboratory-based models like MELD plus Lille. Although this new score was implemented in an assay platform approved by the US Food and Drug Administration, it is not yet commercially available for use and requires a liver biopsy.

Other Prognostic Factors in Alcoholic Hepatitis

There are several other factors that have been shown to predict outcome in AH. Infections are common in severe AH, with a 12% to 26% prevalence at the time of admission, increasing to 50% with exposure to corticosteroids.[50] Infection-related biomarkers like pretreatment serum lipopolysaccharide, bacterial DNA, high-sensitivity C-reactive protein, and procalcitonin are associated with infection risk and 90-day mortality.[51] The presence of SIRS at admission, with or without infection, predicts multiorgan failure (especially acute kidney injury) and early death in severe AH.[48] More recently, Sarin's group in India have identified 9 baseline urinary metabolites like acetyl-L-carnitine that are linked to mitochondrial functions and are significantly associated with pretreatment response to corticosteroids and short-term survival.[52] The same investigators have also reported that the molecular ellipticity of the albumin–bilirubin complex is associated with 3-month survival in severe patients with AH and that the increased loading of bilirubin on albumin could explain the decreased albumin function.[53] Further study is required to validate these findings.

LONGER TERM PROGNOSIS IN ALCOHOLIC HEPATITIS

Whereas short-term prognosis depends on recovery of liver function, in patients surviving beyond 6 months, abstinence from alcohol is the main driver of outcome in patients with severe AH.[54,55] Improvement in long-term survival after severe AH should include secondary prevention strategies to promote complete alcohol abstinence.

Moderate Alcoholic Hepatitis

Patients with moderate AH, defined as an MDF of less than 32 and/or a MELD score of less than 19 but meeting minimal consensus criteria for AH, are being targeted by several intervention studies in the U01 NIAAA Alcoholic Hepatitis Consortia (discussed elsewhere in this article). Moderate AH has been defined as an MDF of less than 32 or a MELD score of less than 19 (discussed elsewhere in this article), in which the short-term (28 days) mortality risk is low (10%–15%), but still significant.[56] Thus, therapies targeting this form of AH are needed and likely more feasible than severe AH. There are safety concerns of potential study drugs in cholestatic livers of severe patients with AH at risk of infection. The phase II trial of the caspase inhibitor emricasan in severe AH was terminated owing to toxicity concerns from high systemic drug levels.[57] The FXR agonist obeticholic acid, approved for primary biliary cholangitis, was recently issued a boxed warning by the US Food and Drug Administration for deaths linked to inappropriate dosing in patients with hepatic impairment (Child class B or C or patients with prior hepatic decompensation). Although even patients with moderate AH may meet these criteria, a highly anticipated phase II trial in moderate AH is currently on hold.[58]

MEDICAL THERAPIES FOR ALCOHOLIC HEPATITIS
Beneficial Therapies

Abstinence
Abstinence from alcohol is the cornerstone of AH treatment. Continued alcohol use in the setting of AH results in increased rates of variceal bleeding, ascites, hepatic encephalopathy, hepatocellular carcinoma, and death.[59–62] Therefore, all patients with AH are advised to establish and maintain lifelong abstinence. The roles of treatments in controlling craving for alcohol or of psychotherapies in supporting abstinence have not been established for in patients with or recovering from AH. Based on other forms of ALD, for which there are also a paucity of good evidence, patient-tailored psychotherapies are recommended once the patient has achieved sufficient health to participate.

Nutrition
Nearly all patients with severe AH and underlying cirrhosis have significant protein–calorie malnutrition. Achieving adequate nutrition can be difficult for patients with severe AH, especially in those with hepatic encephalopathy, tense ascites, and/or lactulose-related ileus. Enteral nutrition via a nasogastric tube is sometimes considered, although good data to support it are few.[63] Passage of a nasogastric tube is generally safe and does not seem to be a risk factor for variceal hemorrhage.[64]

Enteral nutrition may also play a role in reducing bacterial translocation in the gut by maintaining gut barrier function that may decrease the incidence of infections.[65] In a small, multicenter, randomized, prospective Spanish study, enteral nutrition (2000 kcal/d) was compared with prednisolone for 28 days, and similar rates of survival were observed.[66] A follow-up study was then performed, a multicenter, randomized, controlled trial comparing 2 arms—the intensive group, which received intensive enteral nutrition plus methylprednisolone, and the control group that received conventional nutrition plus methylprednisolone.[67] In the intensive group, enteral nutrition of a proprietary formula (1.5 kcal/mL and 7.5 g protein/100 mL) was given via a nasogastric tube for 14 days based on weight (1 L/d if <60 kg, 1.5 L/d if 60–90 kg, or 2 L/d if >90 kg). Intention-to-treat analysis showed no additional survival benefit of nutrition, although patients with a daily calorie intake of less than 21.5 kcal/kg/d had higher mortality at 6 months (65.8%; 95% confidence interval, 48.8–78.4) than those with higher intake. Given these data, adequate and consistent enteral nutrition of greater than 21.5 kcal/kg/d should be given to patients with severe AH.

Corticosteroids
Corticosteroids are the most extensively studied intervention in AH with more than 20 clinical trials that date back more than 4 decades.[5] The heterogeneity and lack of power of these small trials to detect differences in outcome led to years of controversy regarding the utility of corticosteroids in AH. Decreasing mortality of patients with severe AH over time has further compounded the issue. Two Cochrane metaanalyses were conflicted; one reported that corticosteroids decreased 1-month mortality in AH only when severe (DF $\geq$32) or in patients with hepatic encephalopathy.[68,69] A gold standard metaanalysis of combined individual data of 5 randomized, controlled trials with 418 patients confirmed the efficacy of corticosteroids in severe AH.[70] The

arm receiving corticosteroids (n = 221) had higher 28-day survival rates than the placebo arm (n = 197; 80% vs 66%). This finding represented a 30% relative risk reduction with a number needed to treat of 5 (ie, 5 patients need to be treated to avert 1 death at 28 days). In the latest iteration of this metaanalysis, which included more pentoxifylline trial data to reduce bias, corticosteroid treatment significantly reduced mortality at 28 days compared with placebo (hazard ratio, 0.64; 95% confidence interval, 0.48–0.86), representing a 36% risk reduction.[71]

The largest randomized controlled trial in severe AH is the Steroids or Pentoxifylline for Alcoholic Hepatitis (STOPAH) trial, a multicenter, double-blind, randomized trial conducted in 65 hospitals across the United Kingdom with a 2 × 2 factorial design to evaluate the effect of treatment with prednisolone or pentoxifylline on 28-day survival rates over 3 years.[72] The study did not demonstrate a statistically significant survival benefit at 28 days in patients receiving prednisolone compared with placebo (odds ratio, 0.72; 95% confidence interval, 0.52–1.01; $P = .06$). However, on a post hoc multivariable analysis, prednisolone were associated with improved 28-day survival (odds ratio, 0.609; $P = .015$), but not at 90 days or 1 year. The absence of liver biopsy confirmation and lower than expected mortality in the placebo groups likely confounded the study results. The lack of liver biopsy confirmation of AH may have diluted the study population by including subjects without AH, thereby diminishing the study's power. The rates of infection (11%), acute kidney injury (approximately 3%), and overall mortality (16%) were also considerably lower than expected based on prior studies despite high risk scores (mean DF, 62.6; MELD, 21; GAHS, 8). These issues likely confounded the study results despite its optimal study design and large size. The inclusion of patients with acute kidney injury up to a serum creatinine of 5.7 mg/dL (although most were well below this level) and the allowance of terlipressin may have impacted the benefit of pentoxifylline (discussed elsewhere in this article). The STOPAH trial, taken together with the previously discussed evidence, offers support for the recommendation for using prednisolone 40 mg/d for 28 days to improve short-term survival in patients with severe AH (DF ≥32 and without contraindications), with response to treatment assessed using the Lille score.

Clinical management of severe alcoholic hepatitis

Providers are often reticent to start patients with severe AH on corticosteroids owing to side effects and infection risk. There is a significant overlap between the clinical presentations of AH and sepsis. Fever, tachycardia and tachypnea, leukocytosis, altered mental status, abdominal pain, and distension often accompany severe AH. These shared features with SIRS present clinical uncertainty.

Upon admission, providers should obtain blood, urine, ascitic fluid cultures (if possible), chest radiographs, and noncontrast abdominal imaging (eg, ultrasound examination with Doppler), and should avoid empiric antibiotics and nephrotoxic agents. Corticosteroids should be started if a clinical diagnosis of severe AH is made and if cultures are negative at 24 to 48 hours with a low clinical suspicion of infection and a lack of other contraindications (**Fig. 1**). Furthermore, when cultures reveal an infection, corticosteroids may be started after 48 hours of treatment with appropriate antibiotics and clinical stability because this strategy enables recovery of liver function, protection against future infection, and improvement of survival.[50] Although there have been reports of frequent fungal infections resulting in high mortality, particularly *Aspergillus* species, in patients with AH who are treated with corticosteroids in Europe, France, and Belgium, this has not been reported elsewhere in Europe or the United States.[73,74]

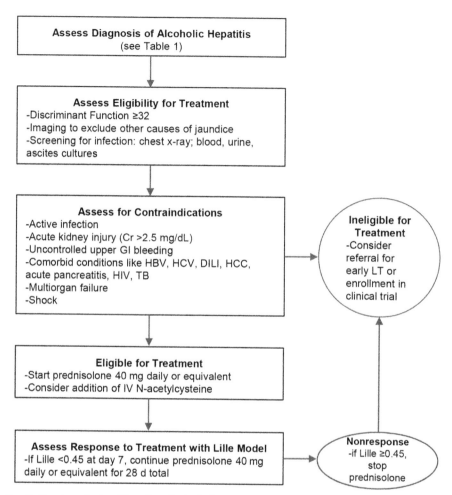

Fig. 1. Treatment algorithm for alcoholic hepatitis. Cr, creatinine; DILI, drug-induced liver injury; GI, gastrointestinal; HBV, hepatitis B virus; HCC, hepatocellular carcinoma; HCV, hepatitis C virus; HIV, human immunodeficiency virus; IV, intravenous; LT, liver transplantation; TB, tuberculosis.

Patients with severe AH are at high risk for acute kidney injury owing to the hepatorenal syndrome. The prognostic significance of the hepatorenal syndrome in AH is reflected in the inclusion of serum creatinine or urea in the previously mentioned prognostic scores. Careful surveillance for this dreaded complication and contraindication to corticosteroids allows for early treatment with intravenous albumin and vasoconstrictors.[75]

Gastrointestinal bleeding (GIB) has been an exclusion criterion for many clinical trials in AH. In a retrospective study of 105 patients with biopsy-proven AH, 55% presented with GIB and the remainder did not.[76] Both groups were given prednisolone; GIB patients started at a mean of 5 days after the bleeding episode (mostly variceal hemorrhage). GIB patients had a lower incidence of infections, likely owing to prophylactic antibiotics, but there were no differences in survival at 1, 3, and 6 months between the 2 groups. This study suggests that GIB is not an absolute contraindication for corticosteroids and that, after control of GIB, prednisolone can be given safely.

Just as there is a minimum threshold at which corticosteroids are useful (DF $\geq$32), a therapeutic ceiling (DF >54) has been posited beyond which medical therapies aimed at decreasing the inflammatory cascade may cause more harm than benefit. The evidence for this is a commonly cited study of protein–calorie malnutrition in US veterans with AH.[77] However, this study was not powered to examine mortality differences at a DF threshold of 54, nor have subsequent studies substantiated this observation. For example, 5 recent studies of corticosteroids in severe AH had a median DF ranging from 54 to 71 with similar rates of mortality.[12,50,72,78,79] Consequently, corticosteroids should not be withheld on the basis of this maximum threshold alone. Nonetheless, a DF of greater than 54 suggests the need to thoroughly assess the patient for undiagnosed infection and/or SIRS before starting corticosteroids.

Potentially beneficial therapies

N-Acetylcysteine N-Acetylcysteine (NAC) reconstitutes glutathione reserves to reduce oxidative stress in mouse models of AH.[80] Intravenous NAC in combination with prednisolone compared with prednisolone plus intravenous placebo was studied in a multicenter, randomized, controlled trial in France.[78] The dosing of NAC was similar to that used in patients with acetaminophen toxicity, but with the 16-hour maintenance dose extended to a total of 5 days. The prednisolone/NAC arm showed an improved 1-month survival compared with prednisolone/placebo (8% vs 24%; P = .006), although this benefit was not seen at 3 or 6 months. The infection rate and mortality attributable to the hepatorenal syndrome were lower in the prednisolone/NAC arm. Because 6-month mortality was the primary endpoint, the study was considered a negative trial for this combination therapy. Because the STOPAH trial demonstrated that corticosteroids reduce mortality in AH only at 1 month, the additional benefit of NAC is promising and deserves further study.

Granulocyte-colony stimulating factor Granulocyte-colony stimulating factor (G-CSF) mobilizes hematopoietic stem cells, induces liver regeneration, and improves survival in experimental models.[81] Two small, randomized, controlled trials of biopsy-proven alcoholic steatohepatitis and cirrhosis demonstrated that 5 days of G-CSF in the treatment arm mobilized CD34$^+$ cells (marker of hematopoietic stem cells), increased hepatocyte growth factor, and induced hepatic progenitor cells to proliferate within 7 days.[82] Subsequent trials of G-CSF in alcohol- and hepatitis B virus-related ACLF in Asia demonstrated an additional benefit of improving liver function and survival with G-CSF at 2 and 3 months, respectively.[83,84] A recent randomized pilot study of 46 patients in India with severe AH receiving pentoxifylline plus G-CSF for 5 days compared outcomes with pentoxifylline alone.[85] There was a significant decrease in the Child-Pugh, MELD, and DF scores and mortality at 90 days in the G-CSF arm. This potential therapy for severe AH is intriguing given its promotion of hepatic regeneration rather than abrogation of inflammation. However, the origin of functional hepatic progenitor cells (eg, liver, peripheral blood) leading to regeneration remains under debate.[86] The data for G-CSF are encouraging but require more study (including cohorts outside of Asia) before wider clinical use can be recommended.

Metadoxine and fecal microbiota transplantation Small pilot studies of the antioxidant metadoxine and fecal microbiota transplantation have also reported improved liver function and survival in patients with severe AH that require verification.[87,88]

Therapies lacking benefit

Pentoxifylline Pentoxifylline is a xanthine derivative that weakly mitigates production of tumor necrosis factor alpha in vitro. Because tumor necrosis factor-α has been proposed to play a major role in the pathogenesis of AH, pentoxifylline was seen as a potential treatment for AH.[89] This finding was further supported by a single randomized, controlled trial comparing pentoxifylline with placebo in patients with severe AH (DF >32), in which the pentoxifylline group showed decreased inpatient mortality and a lower incidence of the hepatorenal syndrome.[90] Subsequent studies have failed to confirm the mortality benefit. A Cochrane metaanalysis reporting on 5 clinical trials of pentoxifylline in severe AH concluded that pentoxifylline could not be supported or rejected for treating AH.[91] Two trials in France failed to show a benefit of pentoxifylline as either a rescue agent in patients who had failed prednisolone (as assessed by Lille score on day 7) or in combination with prednisolone compared with prednisolone alone.[12,92] Furthermore, the STOPAH trial failed to demonstrate any benefit of pentoxifylline over placebo.

Other therapies Well-publicized clinical trials of tumor necrosis factor-α inhibitors infliximab and etanercept in severe AH were terminated early owing to infection-related mortality in the treatment arm.[93] Extracorporeal cellular therapy was studied in a multinational, prospective trial that did not demonstrate survival benefit compared with standard of care.[94] Older trials of various agents, including antioxidants like S-adenosylmethionine and vitamins E, insulin and glucagon, and oxandrolone and propylthiouracil, have failed to demonstrate improvement in survival.[95,96]

Future treatments The overlapping pathophysiology of alcoholic steatohepatitis with nonalcoholic steatohepatitis provides the opportunity for future repurposing of the more imminent treatments being developed for nonalcoholic steatohepatitis. A major initiative from the National Institute on Alcohol Abuse and Alcoholism has supported large, multiinstitutional consortia with the task of identifying new therapeutic targets and performing early phase clinical studies to develop and test new treatments for AH. A review of these rational and targeted potential therapies has been published.[97] The agents attempt to influence different pathophysiologic mechanisms in AH, including disrupted gut–barrier function leading to bacterial and endotoxin translocation, innate immune system activation in the liver, and hepatocellular apoptosis, necrosis, and injury.

REFERENCES

1. Lucey MR, Mathurin P, Morgan TR. Alcoholic hepatitis. N Engl J Med 2009; 360(26):2758–69.
2. Asrani SK, Kamath PS, Pedersen R, et al. Liver related mortality in the US is underestimated. Hepatology 2010;52(2):408–10.
3. Naveau S, Giraud V, Borotto E, et al. Excess weight risk factor for alcoholic liver disease. Hepatology 1997;25(1):108–11.
4. Crabb DW. Pathogenesis of alcoholic liver disease: newer mechanisms of injury. Keio J Med 1999;48:184–8.
5. O'Shea RS, Dasarathy S, McCullough AJ, Practice guideline committee of the American association for the study of liver diseases; practice parameters committee of the American College of Gastroenterology. Alcoholic liver disease. Hepatology 2010;51(1):307–28 [Review. No abstract available].
6. Allen JP, Wurst FM, Thon N, et al. Assessing the drinking status of liver transplant patients with alcoholic liver disease. Liver Transpl 2013;19(4):369–76.

7. Stockwell T, Zhao J, Macdonald S. Who under-reports their alcohol consumption in telephone surveys and by how much? An application of the 'yesterday method' in a national Canadian substance use survey. Addiction 2014;109(10):1657–66.

8. Hope A. Dublin: health service executive; 2009. A standard drink in Ireland: what strength? Available at: www.lenus.ie/hse/handle/10147/80600. Accessed October 4, 2018.

9. Feunekes GI, van 't Veer P, van Staveren WA, et al. Alcohol intake assessment: the sober facts. Am J Epidemiol 1999;150(1):105–12.

10. What's a "standard" drink? Rethinking drinking. Available at: http://rethinkingdrinking.niaaa.nih.gov/whatcountsdrink/whatsastandarddrink.asp. Accessed October 4, 2018.

11. Available at: https://www.centeronaddiction.org/addiction-research/reports/national-survey-primary-care-physicians-patients-substance-abuse. Accessed October 4, 2018.

12. Mathurin P, Louvet A, Duhamel A, et al. Prednisolone with vs without pentoxifylline and survival of patients with severe alcoholic hepatitis: a randomized clinical trial. JAMA 2013;310(10):1033–41.

13. Dunn W, Angulo P, Sanderson S, et al. Utility of a new model to diagnose an alcohol basis for steatohepatitis. Gastroenterology 2006;131(4):1057–63.

14. Hamid R, Forrest EH. Is histology required for the diagnosis of alcoholic hepatitis? A review of published randomised controlled trials. Gut 2011;60(suppl 1):A233.

15. Elphick DA, Dube AK, McFarlane E, et al. Spectrum of liver histology in presumed decompensated alcoholic liver disease. Am J Gastroenterol 2007;102(4):780–8.

16. Mathurin P. Interet de la biopsie hepatique pour la selection des sujets suspects d'hepatite alcoolique aigue. Journees francophones d'hepatologie et de pathologies digestives. Gastroenterol Clin Biol 1992;16:A231.

17. Ramond MJ, Poynard T, Rueff B, et al. A randomized trial of prednisolone in patients with severe alcoholic hepatitis. N Engl J Med 1992;326(8):507–12.

18. Mookerjee RP, Lackner C, Stauber R, et al. The role of liver biopsy in the diagnosis and prognosis of patients with acute deterioration of alcoholic cirrhosis. J Hepatol 2011;55(5):1103–11.

19. Dhanda AD, Collins PL, McCune CA. Is liver biopsy necessary in the management of alcoholic hepatitis? World J Gastroenterol 2013;19(44):7825–9.

20. Kryger P, Schlichting P, Dietrichson O, et al. The accuracy of the clinical diagnosis in acute hepatitis and alcoholic liver disease. Clinical versus morphological diagnosis. Scand J Gastroenterol 1983;18:691–6.

21. Altamirano J, Miquel R, Katoonizadeh A, et al. A histologic scoring system for prognosis of patients with alcoholic hepatitis. Gastroenterology 2014;146:1231–9.e1-6.

22. Popper H, Thung SN, Gerber MA. Pathology of alcoholic liver diseases. Semin Liver Dis 1981;1:203–16.

23. Roth NC, Saberi B, Macklin J, et al. Prediction of histologic alcoholic hepatitis based on clinical presentation limits the need for liver biopsy. Hepatol Commun 2017;1(10):1070–84.

24. Moreau R, Arroyo V. Acute-on-chronic liver failure: a new clinical entity. Clin Gastroenterol Hepatol 2015;13(5):836–41.

25. Katoonizadeh A, Laleman W, Verslype C, et al. Early features of acute-on-chronic alcoholic liver failure: a prospective cohort study. Gut 2010;59(11):1561–9.

26. Sarin SK, Kumar A, Almeida JA, et al. Acute-on-chronic liver failure: consensus recommendations of the Asian Pacific association for the study of the liver (APASL). Hepatol Int 2009;3(1):269–82.

27. Gelsi E, Dainese R, Truchi R, et al. Effect of detoxification on liver stiffness assessed by Fibroscan® in alcoholic patients. Alcohol Clin Exp Res 2011;35(3): 566–70.

28. Thiele M, Detlefsen S, Sevelsted Møller L, et al. Transient and 2-dimensional shear-wave elastography provide comparable assessment of alcoholic liver fibrosis and cirrhosis. Gastroenterology 2016;150(1):123–33.

29. Thiele M, Madsen BS, Hansen JF, et al. Accuracy of the enhanced liver fibrosis test vs FibroTest, elastography, and indirect markers in detection of advanced fibrosis in patients with alcoholic liver disease. Gastroenterology 2018;154(5): 1369–79.

30. Bissonnette J, Altamirano J, Devue C, et al. A prospective study of the utility of plasma biomarkers to diagnose alcoholic hepatitis. Hepatology 2017;66(2): 555–63.

31. Papastergiou V, Tsochatzis EA, Pieri G, et al. Nine scoring models for short-term mortality in alcoholic hepatitis: cross-validation in a biopsy-proven cohort. Aliment Pharmacol Ther 2014;39(7):721–32.

32. Lafferty H, Stanley AJ, Forrest EH. The management of alcoholic hepatitis: a prospective comparison of scoring systems. Aliment Pharmacol Ther 2013;38(6): 603–10.

33. Maddrey WC, Boitnott JK, Bedine MS, et al. Corticosteroid therapy of alcoholic hepatitis. Gastroenterology 1978;75(2):193–9.

34. Bellest L, Eschwège V, Poupon R, et al. A modified international normalized ratio as an effective way of prothrombin time standardization in hepatology. Hepatology 2007;46(2):528–34.

35. Battish R, Shah H, Sherker AH. Does selection of prothrombin time normal value alter prognosis according to Maddrey discriminant function in alcoholic hepatitis? Gastroenterology 2010;138(5 suppl 1):S-806.

36. Mathurin P, Abdelnour M, Ramond MJ, et al. Early change in bilirubin levels is an important prognostic factor in severe alcoholic hepatitis treated with prednisolone. Hepatology 2003;38(6):1363–9.

37. Louvet A, Naveau S, Abdelnour M, et al. The Lille model: a new tool for therapeutic strategy in patients with severe alcoholic hepatitis treated with steroids. Hepatology 2007;45(6):1348–54.

38. Mathurin P, O'Grady J, Carithers RL, et al. Corticosteroids improve short-term survival in patients with severe alcoholic hepatitis: meta-analysis of individual patient data. Gut 2011;60(2):255–60.

39. Garcia-Saenz-de-Sicilia M, Duvoor C, Altamirano J, et al. A day-4 Lille model predicts response to corticosteroids and mortality in severe alcoholic hepatitis. Am J Gastroenterol 2017;112(2):306–15.

40. Altamirano J, Fagundes C, Dominguez M, et al. Acute kidney injury is an early predictor of mortality for patients with alcoholic hepatitis. Clin Gastroenterol Hepatol 2012;10(1):65–71.e3.

41. Dunn W, Jamil LH, Brown LS, et al. MELD accurately predicts mortality in patients with alcoholic hepatitis. Hepatology 2005;41(2):353–8.

42. Srikureja W, Kyulo NL, Runyon BA, et al. MELD score is a better prognostic model than Child-Turcotte-Pugh score or discriminant function score in patients with alcoholic hepatitis. J Hepatol 2005;42(5):700–6.

43. Bajaj JS, O'Leary JG, Reddy KR, et al. NACSELD. Second infections independently increase mortality in hospitalized patients with cirrhosis: the North American Consortium for the Study of End-Stage Liver Disease (NACSELD) experience. Hepatology 2012;56(6):2328–35.

44. Forrest EH, Evans CD, Stewart S, et al. Analysis of factors predictive of mortality in alcoholic hepatitis and derivation and validation of the Glasgow alcoholic hepatitis score. Gut 2005;54(8):1174–9.

45. Forrest EH, Morris AJ, Stewart S, et al. The Glasgow alcoholic hepatitis score identifies patients who may benefit from corticosteroids. Gut 2007;56(12):1743–6.

46. Dominguez M, Rincón D, Abraldes JG, et al. A new scoring system for prognostic stratification of patients with alcoholic hepatitis. Am J Gastroenterol 2008;103(11): 2747–56.

47. Louvet A, Labreuche J, Artru F, et al. Combining data from liver disease scoring systems better predicts outcomes of patients with alcoholic hepatitis. Gastroenterology 2015;149(2):398–406.e8.

48. Michelena J, Altamirano J, Abraldes JG, et al. Systemic inflammatory response and serum lipopolysaccharide levels predict multiple organ failure and death in alcoholic hepatitis. Hepatology 2015;62(3):762–72.

49. Trépo E, Goossens N, Fujiwara N, et al. Combination of gene expression signature and model for end-stage liver disease score predicts survival of patients with severe alcoholic hepatitis. Gastroenterology 2018;154(4):965–75.

50. Louvet A, Wartel F, Castel H, et al. Infection in patients with severe alcoholic hepatitis treated with steroids: early response to therapy is the key factor. Gastroenterology 2009;137(2):541–8.

51. Vergis N, Atkinson SR, Knapp S, et al. In patients with severe alcoholic hepatitis, prednisolone increases susceptibility to infection and infection-related mortality, and is associated with high circulating levels of bacterial DNA. Gastroenterology 2017;152(5):1068–77.e4.

52. Maras JS, Das S, Sharma S, et al. Baseline urine metabolic phenotype in patients with severe alcoholic hepatitis and its association with outcome. Hepatol Commun 2018;2(6):628–43.

53. Das S, Maras JS, Maiwall R, et al. Molecular ellipticity of circulating albumin-bilirubin complex associates with mortality in patients with severe alcoholic hepatitis. Clin Gastroenterol Hepatol 2018;16(8):1322–32.e4.

54. Louvet A, Labreuche J, Artru F, et al. Main drivers of outcome differ between short term and long term in severe alcoholic hepatitis: a prospective study. Hepatology 2017;66:1464–73.

55. Altamirano J, López-Pelayo H, Michelena J, et al. Alcohol abstinence in patients surviving an episode of alcoholic hepatitis: prediction and impact on long-term survival. Hepatology 2017;66(6):1842–53.

56. Kulkarni K, Tran T, Medrano M, et al. The role of the discriminant factor in the assessment and treatment of alcoholic hepatitis. J Clin Gastroenterol 2004; 38(5):453–9.

57. Available at: https://clinicaltrials.gov/ct2/show/NCT01912404. Accessed October 4, 2018.

58. Peeraphatdit TB, Simonetto DA, Shah VH. Exploring new treatment paradigms for alcoholic hepatitis by extrapolating from NASH and cholestasis. J Hepatol 2018; 69(2):275–7.

59. Lucey MR, Connor JT, Boyer TD, et al. Alcohol consumption by cirrhotic subjects: patterns of use and effects on liver function. Am J Gastroenterol 2008;103: 1698–706.

60. Verrill C, Markham H, Templeton A, et al. Alcohol-related cirrhosis—early abstinence is a key factor in prognosis, even in the most severe cases. Addiction 2009;104:768–74.

61. Potts JR, Goubet S, Heneghan MA, et al. Determinants of long-term outcome in severe alcoholic hepatitis. Aliment Pharmacol Ther 2013;38:584–95.

62. Dumortier JEROM, Dharancy SEB, Cannesson AEL, et al. Recurrent alcoholic cirrhosis in severe alcoholic relapse after liver transplantation: a frequent and serious complication. Am J Gastroenterol 2015;110:1–7.

63. Chan LN. To hold (enteral feeding) or not to hold: that is the question; a commentary and tutorial. Pract Gastroenterol 2012;36(1):13–21.

64. Tai M, Razlan H, Goh K, et al. Short term nasogastric versus oral feeding in hospitalised patients with advanced cirrhosis: A randomised trial. e-SPEN 2011; 2011(6):e242–7.

65. MacFie J. Enteral versus parenteral nutrition: the significance of bacterial translocation and gut-barrier function. Nutrition 2000;16(7–8):606–11.

66. Cabre E, Gonzalez-Huix F, Abad-Lacruz A, et al. Effect of total enteral nutrition on the short-term outcome of severely malnourished cirrhotics. A randomized controlled trial. Gastroenterology 1990;98(3):715–20.

67. Moreno C, Trepo E, Louvet A, et al. Impact of intensive enteral nutrition in association with corticosteroids in the treatment of severe alcoholic hepatitis: a multicenter randomized controlled trial. Hepatology 2014;60(4):269A.

68. Christensen E, Gluud C. Glucocorticoids are ineffective in alcoholic hepatitis: a meta-analysis adjusting for confounding variables. Gut 1995;37(1):113–8.

69. Rambaldi A, Saconato HH, Christensen E, et al. Systematic review: glucocorticosteroids for alcoholic hepatitis—a Cochrane Hepato-Biliary Group systematic review with meta-analyses and trial sequential analyses of randomized clinical trials. Aliment Pharmacol Ther 2008;27(12):1167–78.

70. Mathurin P, O'Grady J, Carithers RL, et al. Corticosteroids improve 28-day survival in patients with severe alcoholic hepatitis: individual data analysis of the last 5 randomized controlled trials. Hepatology 2008;48:170A.

71. Louvet A, Thursz MR, Kim DJ, et al. Corticosteroids reduce risk of death within 28 days for patients with severe alcoholic hepatitis, compared with pentoxifylline or placebo-a meta-analysis of individual data. Gastroenterology 2018;155(2): 458–68.e8.

72. Thursz MR, Richardson P, Allison M, et al. STOPAH trial. Prednisolone or pentoxifylline for alcoholic hepatitis. N Engl J Med 2015;372(17):1619–28.

73. Gustot T, Maillart E, Bocci M, et al. Invasive aspergillosis in patients with severe alcoholic hepatitis. J Hepatol 2014;60(2):267–74.

74. Parker R, Im G, Jones F, et al. Clinical and microbiological features of infection in alcoholic hepatitis: an international cohort study. J Gastroenterol 2017;52(11): 1192–200.

75. Mathurin P, Lucey MR. Management of alcoholic hepatitis. J Hepatol 2012; 56(Suppl 1):S39–45.

76. Rudler M, Mouri S, Charlotte F, et al. Prognosis of treated severe alcoholic hepatitis in patients with gastrointestinal bleeding. J Hepatol 2015;62(4):816–21.

77. Mendenhall C, Roselle GA, Gartside P, et al. Relationship of protein calorie malnutrition to alcoholic liver disease: a reexamination of data from two veterans administration cooperative studies. Alcohol Clin Exp Res 1995;19(3):635–41.

78. Nguyen-Khac E, Thevenot T, Piquet MA, et al, AAH-NAC Study Group. Glucocorticoids plus N-acetylcysteine in severe alcoholic hepatitis. N Engl J Med 2011; 365(19):1781–9.

79. Stewart S, Prince M, Bassendine M, et al. A randomized trial of antioxidant therapy alone or with corticosteroids in acute alcoholic hepatitis. J Hepatol 2007; 47(2):277–83.

80. Wang AL, Wang JP, Wang H, et al. A dual effect of N-acetylcysteine on acute ethanol-induced liver damage in mice. Hepatol Res 2006;34(3):199–206.
81. Spahr L, Lambert JF, Rubbia-Brandt L, et al. Granulocyte-colony stimulating factor induces proliferation of hepatic progenitors in alcoholic steatohepatitis: a randomized trial. Hepatology 2008;48(1):221–9.
82. Di Campli C, Zocco MA, Saulnier N, et al. Safety and efficacy profile of G-CSF therapy in patients with acute on chronic liver failure. Dig Liver Dis 2007; 39(12):1071–6.
83. Garg V, Garg H, Khan A, et al. Granulocyte colony-stimulating factor mobilizes CD34(+) cells and improves survival of patients with acute-on-chronic liver failure. Gastroenterology 2012;142(3):505–12.e1.
84. Duan XZ, Liu FF, Tong JJ, et al. Granulocyte-colony stimulating factor therapy improves survival in patients with hepatitis B virus-associated acute-on-chronic liver failure. World J Gastroenterol 2013;19(7):1104–10.
85. Singh V, Sharma AK, Narasimhan RL, et al. Granulocyte colony-stimulating factor in severe alcoholic hepatitis: a randomized pilot study. Am J Gastroenterol 2014; 109(9):1417–23.
86. Popp FC, Piso P, Schlitt HJ, et al. Therapeutic potential of bone marrow stem cells for liver diseases. Curr Stem Cell Res Ther 2006;1(3):411–8.
87. Philips CA, Pande A, Shasthry SM, et al. Healthy donor fecal microbiota transplantation in steroid-ineligible severe alcoholic hepatitis: a pilot study. Clin Gastroenterol Hepatol 2017;15(4):600–2.
88. Higuera-de la Tijera F, Servín-Caamaño AI, Serralde-Zúñiga AE, et al. Metadoxine improves the three- and six-month survival rates in patients with severe alcoholic hepatitis. World J Gastroenterol 2015;21(16):4975–85.
89. McClain CJ, Cohen DA. Increased tumor necrosis factor production by monocytes in alcoholic hepatitis. Hepatology 1989;9(3):349–51.
90. Akriviadis E, Botla R, Briggs W, et al. Pentoxifylline improves short-term survival in severe acute alcoholic hepatitis: a double-blind, placebo-controlled trial. Gastroenterology 2000;119(6):1637–48.
91. Whitfield K, Rambaldi A, Wetterslev J, et al. Pentoxifylline for alcoholic hepatitis. Cochrane Database Syst Rev 2009;(4):CD007339.
92. Louvet A, Diaz E, Dharancy S, et al. Early switch to pentoxifylline in patients with severe alcoholic hepatitis is inefficient in non-responders to corticosteroids. J Hepatol 2008;48(3):465–70.
93. Spahr L, Rubbia-Brandt L, Frossard JL, et al. Combination of steroids with infliximab or placebo in severe alcoholic hepatitis: a randomized controlled pilot study. J Hepatol 2002;37(4):448–55.
94. Thompson J, Jones N, Al-Khafaji A, et al. Extracorporeal cellular therapy (ELAD) in severe alcoholic hepatitis: a multinational, prospective, controlled, randomized trial. Liver Transpl 2018;24(3):380–93.
95. Bjelakovic G, Gluud LL, Nikolova D, et al. Antioxidant supplements for liver diseases. Cochrane Database Syst Rev 2011;(16):CD007749.
96. Phillips M, Curtis H, Portmann B, et al. Antioxidants versus corticosteroids in the treatment of severe alcoholic hepatitis–a randomised clinical trial. J Hepatol 2006;44:784–90.
97. Singal AK, Kamath PS, Gores GJ, et al. Alcoholic hepatitis: current challenges and future directions. Clin Gastroenterol Hepatol 2014;12(4):555–64.

Nutrition in Alcoholic Liver Disease: An Update

Brett Styskel, MD[a], Yamini Natarajan, MD[a],*,
Fasiha Kanwal, MD, MSHS[a,b,c]

KEYWORDS

- Malnutrition • Overnutrition • Undernutrition • Alcoholic liver disease • Cirrhosis
- Alcoholic hepatitis • Albumin

KEY POINTS

- Malnutrition is exceptionally common in patients with alcoholic liver disease, approaching 100% in patients admitted to the hospital for alcoholic hepatitis and in patients with jaundice.
- Nutritional status should be assessed in patients with alcoholic liver disease, and can be done using simple, inexpensive bedside tests such as the subjective global assessment, anthropometry, and handgrip strength.
- Using serum proteins such as albumin, prealbumin and transferrin can be misleading owing to decreased synthetic function of the liver and the use of intravenous albumin in patients with liver disease.
- The reasons underlying malnutrition are multifactorial and include caloric intake shifting toward carbohydrates, decreased gastric volume owing to ascites, altered olfactory and gustatory perception, alterations in appetite-related hormones, malabsorption, and potentially altered microbiota.

INTRODUCTION

Malnutrition is a change in body composition owing to disordered nutrition associated with a decrease in function and poor clinical outcomes. Malnutrition can result from overnutrition, undernutrition and inflammatory activity.[1] Patients with alcoholic liver disease (ALD) are at increased risk for malnutrition. In this article, we discuss the

The authors have nothing to disclose.

[a] Section of Gastroenterology and Hepatology, Michael E. DeBakey VA Medical Center, Baylor College of Medicine, Houston, TX 77030, USA; [b] Center for Innovations in Quality, Effectiveness and Safety (IQuESt), Michael E. DeBakey VA Medical Center, Houston, TX 77030, USA; [c] Section of Health Services Research, Department of Medicine, Baylor College of Medicine, Houston, TX 77030, USA
* Corresponding author.
E-mail address: ynataraj@bcm.edu

different methods used to assess malnutrition, prevalence of malnutrition, potential mechanisms underlying malnutrition, and its treatments in patients with ALD.

ASSESSMENT OF MALNUTRITION

There is no gold standard method for assessing malnutrition. Studies have used multiple methods including the subjective global assessment (SGA), anthropometric measurements, serum protein levels, immune function, muscle strength, dry body mass index (BMI), and creatinine–height index (**Table 1**). Of these, the European Society for Clinical Nutrition and Metabolism recommends the SGA, anthropometry, or handgrip strength to assess for malnutrition in patients with ALD.[2]

History and Physical

A detailed history and physical examination can be an important and cost-effective tool to evaluate malnutrition. Components to consider include changes in weight, dietary and alcohol intake, and changes in functional status. A thorough physical examination should evaluate for muscle wasting, edema, ascites, and findings of nutrient deficiencies such as skin changes and neurologic deficits.[3]

Dry BMI has been used to diagnose malnutrition in patients with advanced liver disease. With this method, a patient's height and weight are used to determine ideal BMI. Using ultrasound examination, the severity of ascites is divided into 3 categories (mild, moderate, or severe). In the presence of mild ascites, 5% of the body weight is subtracted, 10% is subtracted for moderate ascites, and 15% is subtracted for severe ascites. This method was found to be an accurate tool to assess for protein–calorie malnutrition using midarm muscle circumference and triceps skinfold thickness as the reference standards.[4–6]

Subjective Global Assessment

The SGA is a survey-based scoring system using questions regarding weight change, dietary intake, gastrointestinal symptoms, functional capacity, metabolic demand, and physical examination components.[3,7] Morgan and colleagues[8] validated the use of the SGA in assessing nutritional status in patients with cirrhosis. When compared with BMI and midarm muscle circumference in 50 patients with cirrhosis, the SGA showed good interobserver agreement for classifying patients as adequately nourished, moderately malnourished, or severely malnourished. Additionally, the SGA showed a significant association with worsening nutritional status and decreased survival.[8]

Anthropometric Measurements

Anthropometric measurements include weight, height, waist circumference, hip circumference, skinfold thickness, and midarm circumference.[6] The benefits of anthropometric measurements include the ease with which they can be performed at the bedside to assess malnutrition in ALD.[5,9,10] Potential drawbacks of anthropometric measurements include decreased accuracy in patients with edema, which is common among patients with cirrhosis.[11,12]

Laboratory Tests

Serum proteins such as albumin, prealbumin, and the international normalized ratio are frequently used to assess protein malnutrition. Although their use is widespread, there are many limitations to these markers. These proteins are synthesized by the liver, so decreased levels may be affected equally by hepatic dysfunction, hepatic

Table 1
Methods to evaluate malnutrition in alcoholic liver disease: Evidence to the support accuracy of the measurement method

Method	Strengths	Weaknesses	Cutoffs	Sensitivity	Specificity	PPV	NPV	Area Under the Curve	Spearman's Correlation	Standard	Cohort	Reference
SGA	Low cost, easily performed at bedside	Subjective							Relative to BMI: r = −0.78 (P < .001) Relative to MAMC: r = −.069 (P < .001)	BMI, MAMC	NA	Morgan et al,[8] 2006
Anthropometric measurements	Low cost, easily performed at bedside	Potential for inaccuracy if edema present	Mid-arm circumference of 28.2 cm in males	81%	90%	97%		0.87; 95% CI, 0.77–0.97		SGA	Cirrhotic (any etiology) preliver transplant patients	Marr et al,[5] 2017
Visceral proteins	Physician familiarity, simple blood test	Decreased liver synthetic function, use of IV albumin limits accuracy										
Handgrip strength	Accurate, objective, easily performed at bedside		Hand grip of <30 kg and MAMC of <23 cm	94%			97%				Detecting body cell mass depletion in patients with end-stage liver disease of any etiology	Singal et al,[23] 2013

(continued on next page)

Table 1
(continued)

Method	Strengths	Weaknesses	Cutoffs	Sensitivity	Specificity	PPV	NPV	Area Under the Curve	Spearman's Correlation	Standard	Cohort	Reference
BMI	Low cost, data readily available	Potential inaccuracy if edema present	Reference values: No ascites, BMI $\leq$22 kg/m². Mild ascites, BMI $\leq$23 kg/m². Tension ascites, BMI $\leq$25 kg/m².	86%	90%			0.78–0.86		MAMC and triceps skinfold thickness	Cirrhosis of any etiology	Moctezuma et al,[6] 2013; Campillo et al,[83] 2006
Dry BMI	Low cost, data readily available	Potential inaccuracy if edema present						0.78; 95% CI, 0.65–0.90		SGA	Cirrhotic (any etiology) in preliver transplant patients	Marr et al,[5] 2017
Creatinine height index	Low cost, data readily available	High prevalence of kidney disease limits its usefulness										

Abbreviations: BMI, body mass index; CI, confidence interval; IV, intravenous; MAMC, mid-arm muscle circumference; NA, not applicable; NPV, negative predictive value; PPV, positive predictive value; SGA, subjective global assessment.

inflammation, and malnutrition. Also, the widespread use of intravenous albumin (after paracentesis, to treat hepatorenal syndrome, etc.) may limit the use of serum albumin as a measure of malnutrition in ALD.[7]

In contrast, serum levels of vitamins such as vitamins A, D, E, and K should be tested in the appropriate clinical contexts (**Table 2**). Macrocytic anemia should prompt testing for vitamin B_{12} and folate deficiency, and microcytic anemia should prompt testing for iron deficiency. Alcohol may directly cause a macrocytosis, which is discussed elsewhere in this article. The creatinine–height index is a commonly used method to estimate muscle mass; the finding of decreased muscle mass can be used as a surrogate for malnutrition. Total muscle mass is estimated by measuring 24-hour urinary creatinine excretion, which is measured as:

1 g of creatinine = 18.5 kg of muscle mass

This method, however, can underestimate muscle mass when creatinine clearance is decreased owing to acute and/or chronic kidney disease.[13]

Ancillary Tests

Immune function, including total lymphocyte count, has also been investigated for its use in assessing malnutrition. Alcohol consumption impairs host defenses.[14–16] The usefulness of this test as an assessment tool in ALD is uncertain, given that there are few studies with small sample sizes.[3,16]

Handgrip strength can be used as a measure of nutritional status in ALD. Handgrip strength is measured using a dynamometer, which measures force output. Decreased handgrip strength is considered a sign of diminished skeletal muscle mass. Available data show that handgrip strength reliably decreases with worsening nutritional status in ALD.[5]

Using the SGA as the reference standard, a recent study compared various bedside malnutrition measurements, including handgrip strength, midarm circumference, and dry BMI. All methods were similarly accurate for assessing malnutrition in patients with cirrhosis.[5] However, in 50 outpatients with cirrhosis, handgrip strength was more accurate than the SGA in predicting suboptimal outcomes.[17] Notable limitations include muscle or nerve injury, diabetes, and variable effort.

Table 2
Clinical features associated with vitamin deficiencies in alcoholic liver disease

Vitamin	Clinical Findings
A	Night blindness, increased fibrosis
B_1 (thiamine)	Wernicke-Korsakoff syndrome, neuropathy, heart failure
B_3	Pellagra
B_6	Rash, glossitis, neuropathy, sideroblastic anemia
B_9	Macrocytic anemia
B_{12}	Macrocytic anemia, neuropathy, weakness
C	Scurvy
D	Decreased bone density/osteoporosis
E	Neurologic deficits, myopathy, immune cell dysfunction

PREVALENCE OF MALNUTRITION IN ALCOHOLIC LIVER DISEASE

Numerous studies have examined the prevalence of malnutrition in ALD. Although these studies used different methods for assessment, all consistently found a high prevalence of malnutrition in patients with ALD. Patients with chronic liver disease of any etiology often experience malnutrition, with reported prevalence ranging from 50% to 90% among patients with cirrhosis.[18–21] The prevalence of malnutrition ranges from 12% to 100% in patients with ALD[22–24] (**Table 3**). Data from a study involving 6 Veterans Administration hospitals evaluating 360 patients with alcoholic hepatitis showed that 100% had some degree of malnutrition based on many modalities of measurement.[25] Additionally, among 536 patients with liver disease who developed jaundice, 100% had some degree of malnutrition. The severity of malnutrition was closely associated with complications of liver disease, including encephalopathy, ascites, hepatorenal syndrome, and overall mortality.[2] These trends have not changed over time. For example, a recent study by Singal and colleagues[23] found that, among 261 patients with alcoholic cirrhosis undergoing transplantation, 84% had malnutrition when assessed with the SGA.

ETIOLOGY OF MALNUTRITION

Two pathways are postulated to contribute to malnutrition in ALD: (1) direct effects of ethanol and (2) downstream effects of advanced liver disease.

Mechanisms Directly Related to Alcohol

Alcohol use can result in malnutrition by several mechanisms. Patients who consume excessive alcohol typically get a large percentage of their total daily calories in the form of carbohydrate (alcohol). This diet is usually lacking in protein, fats, and micronutrients.[26,27] This mismatch increases with increasing severity of liver disease.[25] Alcohol affects DNA methylation via decreased absorption of folate and other pathways (PMID: 24313162). Alcohol, via its byproduct acetaldehyde, impairs skeletal muscle synthesis and increases autophagy.[28–30] Local metabolism of alcohol in skeletal muscle also leads to reactive oxygen species and mitochondrial dysfunction.[31] Nutrient absorption is impaired via alterations in the gut microbiome and gut permeability. Impaired permeability leads to an increased absorption of lipopolysaccharide (endotoxin), creating a proinflammatory state.[32]

Mechanisms Related to Liver Dysfunction

The progression of liver disease may further contribute to malnutrition in ALD. Patients with cirrhosis and ascites (from any etiology, including ALD) commonly experience postprandial fullness caused by decreased gastric volume.[33] Taste and smell may be altered by vitamin A and zinc deficiency,[34–36] and altered levels of glucose, ghrelin, and leptin may affect satiety. All these factors contribute to decreased caloric intake and increased weight loss in ALD and cirrhosis.[37,38]

Many factors may also contribute to malabsorption in patients with cirrhosis, regardless of etiology. A study of small bowel motility and small intestinal bacterial overgrowth in 56 patients with cirrhosis and portal hypertension showed a significantly greater proportion of retrograde individual pressure waves in the proximal duodenum postprandially (49%), when compared with patients with cirrhosis alone (18%), and healthy controls (13%).[39] Further, there was a nonsignificant trend toward small intestinal bacterial overgrowth in patients with cirrhosis and portal hypertension (33%) compared with cirrhosis alone (0%). In addition, some patients may have coexisting chronic pancreatitis, which can play a role in malabsorption.[40]

Table 3
Prevalence of malnutrition in alcoholic liver disease

Author, Year	Patients	Setting	N	Method of Measurement	Key Findings
Mendenhall et al,[25] 1984	Alcohol abuse with alcoholic hepatitis	Inpatient	363	Visceral proteins, immune response to skin tests, creatinine–height index, percent of ideal body weight	100% of patients with liver disease, admitted for alcohol abuse with alcoholic hepatitis
Mendenhall et al,[22] 1995	Alcoholic hepatitis	Inpatient	536	Visceral proteins, immune response to skin tests, creatinine–height index, percent of ideal body weight, skin fold thickness, midarm muscle area, total lymphocyte count grip strength, CD4 count, CD4:CD8 ratio	100% of patients with clinical jaundice
Mendenhall et al,[22] 1995	Alcohol abuse without laboratory evidence of liver injury	Outpatient	43	Visceral proteins, immune response to skin tests, creatinine–height index, percent of ideal body weight, skin fold thickness, midarm muscle area, total lymphocyte count grip strength, CD4 count, CD4:CD8 ratio	62% of patients with alcohol abuse without liver injury had some findings of malnutrition
Singal et al,[23] 2013	Patients with alcoholic cirrhosis undergoing liver transplantation	Inpatient	261	Subjective global assessment	84% of patients undergoing liver transplantation.

In liver disease and cirrhosis, there is a shift in the microbiota toward firmicutes, which affects the metabolism of bile acids in the gut.[41] Alcohol intake accelerates this process, and changes in the bacterial composition of the gut can also have an impact on intestinal and systemic inflammation. Hyperammonemia may also contribute to sarcopenia by inhibiting the mTORC1 pathway.[42] Patients with cirrhosis commonly exhibit a hypermetabolic state.[43,44] Resting energy expenditure is further increased in the presence of neoplasm and ascites.[9]

Socioeconomic factors may also contribute to the high prevalence of malnutrition in ALD. Lower socioeconomic status, which may be more common in patients with ALD than those with liver disease from other etiologies, is a risk factor for a poorly balanced diet deficient in folate, vitamin B_{12}, vitamin B_6, and macronutrients.[9,45,46]

OUTCOMES AND TREATMENT OF MALNUTRITION IN ALCOHOLIC LIVER DISEASE

Malnutrition has a significant impact on patient outcomes, such as mortality and hospitalization, in patients with ALD.[18,47,48] Enteral supplementation in hospitalized and ambulatory patient may lead to improved outcomes. Additionally, studies continue to underscore the importance of nutrition in patients with alcoholic hepatitis and patients before and after liver transplantation. In addition to clinical outcomes, malnutrition has a major negative impact on the cost of hospitalization for patients with ALD. We cover these aspects in the next section.

Outcomes and Treatment of Malnutrition in Patients with Chronic Alcoholic Liver Disease

Despite the high prevalence of malnutrition among patients hospitalized with ALD and its association with increased short-term and long-term mortality, nutritional interventions are underused. A retrospective cohort study found that up to 43% of hospitalized patients with cirrhosis did not receive any assessment for nutritional status, and only one-third of patients with malnutrition and poor caloric intake received nutritional support.[21] Malnourished patients were significantly more likely to die during hospitalization than those with adequate nutrition (24.3% vs 5.3%, respectively). Only 8% of malnourished patients were seen in the outpatient dietician clinic after discharge from the hospital.[21]

Protein–calorie malnutrition has a significant impact on the cost of inpatient care in patients admitted with ALD.[24] In a population-based cross-sectional study including 72,531 hospitalizations with ALD and 287,047 hospitalizations with other alcohol-related diagnoses, the per-patient cost for hospitalizations were more than $3000 higher in patients with ALD than in patients with other alcohol-related disease ($13,543 vs $10,355; $P < .001$). Protein–calorie malnutrition contributed the most to this difference in cost of care.

There are a paucity of data addressing nutritional interventions in outpatients with ALD. In a randomized, controlled trial by Hirsch and colleagues[49] involving 51 ambulatory patients, 26 study patients were given a supplement of 1000 Kcal including 34 g protein, whereas another 25 patients were treated with standard of care (no supplementation). In 1 year, patients treated with nutritional supplementation were hospitalized less frequently than patients without supplementation (23 occasions compared with 35 occasions). The reduction in frequency of hospitalizations was related to a decrease in severe infections in the intervention arm. Notably, 9 patients died during the study; 6 were in the control arm and 3 in the intervention arm ($P = $ NS).

In summary, the available studies show that patients with chronic ALD should be assessed for malnutrition, and physicians should begin nutritional intervention when deficiencies are identified. Efforts should be made to ensure adequate outpatient follow-up.

Outcomes and Treatment of Malnutrition in Patients with Alcoholic Hepatitis

Data from randomized, controlled trials demonstrate the benefits of enteral nutrition in patients with alcoholic hepatitis. A systematic review and metaanalysis of randomized, controlled trials comparing nutritional therapy with placebo or no intervention in patients with cirrhosis of any etiology or alcoholic hepatitis found that nutritional therapy was associated with a statistically significant benefit in multiple clinical outcomes, including the occurrence of hepatic encephalopathy, infection, and mortality.[50] However, all studies had a high risk of bias. Therefore, high-quality data are still needed to confirm these findings and to guide the selection of the type and duration of nutritional support therapy.

One trial also compared nutrition with steroid therapy in patients with alcoholic hepatitis.[51] Patients were randomized to a 2000 kcal/d diet enriched in branched-chain amino acids versus 40 mg/d of oral prednisolone. There was no difference in the mortality rate at 1 month, but the mortality rate at 1 year was significantly lower in the enteral nutrition group compared with the glucocorticoid group. Indeed, the American College of Gastroenterology guidelines on alcoholic hepatitis recommend that all patients with alcoholic hepatitis should be assessed for malnutrition and receive supplementation to meet their caloric needs.[52] Importantly, all patients in the Steroids or Pentoxyfylline for Alcoholic Hepatitis (STOPAH) trial were given nutritional support, reflecting the importance of nutrition in this context.[53]

Outcomes and Treatment of Malnutrition in Patients with Liver Transplantation

Malnutrition is an independent risk factor for the number of days spent in the intensive care unit and the total hospital length of stay in patients awaiting liver transplantation.[18,54] Data are conflicting regarding the effect of malnutrition on patient outcomes after transplantation. One retrospective study of patients with alcoholic cirrhosis undergoing transplantation found excellent 1-year graft and patient survival rates; these outcomes were not associated with nutritional state at the time of transplantation.[23] The study was limited by its retrospective nature and selection bias for transplantation.

MANAGEMENT OF NUTRITIONAL DEFICIENCIES

The treatment of nutrient deficiency in patients with ALD focuses on abstinence from alcohol and managing protein–calorie malnutrition. The assessment and treatment of malnutrition in ALD should also include replacement of macronutrients and micronutrients, including branched chain amino acids, vitamins, and minerals (**Table 4**).

Alcohol Abstinence

In patients with chronic liver disease, meeting daily caloric intake is a frequent problem. Abstinent patients have a higher caloric intake compared with those with ongoing alcohol use,[45] and abstinence may boost the beneficial effects of nutritional support on host defenses.[55] Abstinence may have other beneficial effects on malnutrition that have not been fully characterized.

Table 4
Prevalence, testing, and treatment for specific deficiencies

	Prevalence	Testing	Treatment
Calories	See **Table 3**	Evaluate in all patients with ALD	35–40 kcal/g/kg BW/d in patients with liver cirrhosis
Protein	See **Table 3**	Evaluate in all patients with ALD	1.2–1.5 g/kg BW/d in patients with liver cirrhosis
Vitamin A	Prevalence data limited	Test in patients with findings suggestive of deficiency	Treat on a case-by-case basis; use caution in patients who continue to ingest alcohol, which can potentiate hepatotoxicity
Vitamin B$_{12}$	25% of hospitalized patients with chronic alcohol consumption	Test in patients with findings suggestive of deficiency	Replete and monitor B$_{12}$ levels if deficiency exists
Folate	80% of hospitalized patients with chronic alcohol consumption	Test in patients with findings suggestive of deficiency	Replete and monitor folate levels if deficiency exists
Vitamin D	86.5% of patients with cirrhosis, 49.0% in patients with liver disease without cirrhosis	High prevalence in chronic liver disease (86.3%); although limited data exists, can consider screening	Single large dose of ergocalciferol compared with cholecalciferol may be more effective in alcoholic liver disease
Vitamin E	Prevalence data are limited	Test in patients with findings suggestive of deficiency	Treat if deficiency exists; no proven benefit of supplementation in absence of deficiency
Zinc	83% of patients with cirrhosis	Test in patients with findings suggestive of deficiency	Zinc supplementation improved Child-Pugh class at 3 mo in alcoholic cirrhosis; further studies are needed but, one can consider supplementation

Energy and Protein Intake

The European Society for Clinical Nutrition and Metabolism recommends energy intake of 35 to 40 kcal/kg body weight per day, with a recommended protein intake of 1.2 to 1.5 g/kg body weight per day in patients with cirrhosis regardless of etiology.[2]

Vitamin A

ALD is associated with low levels of vitamin A; the level of deficiency correlates with the severity of liver disease.[56–58] The mechanism for such disturbances in vitamin A includes the shared metabolic pathway between ethanol metabolism and retinoid compounds. The biochemical metabolism of ethanol and retinol both involve alcohol dehydrogenase subtypes.[59] Vitamin A deficiency can lead to night blindness and hypogonadism, both of which have been described in patients who consume alcohol.[57] Vitamin A has also been implicated in hypogeusia and insomnia in patients with liver disease, which may worsen alcohol-induced liver injury and promote carcinogenesis.[34,60] Paradoxically, in patients with ALD who continue to ingest alcohol, the hepatotoxicity of vitamin A is amplified by alcohol use, and vitamin A excess in patients with ALD may promote carcinogenesis.[60] Thus, vitamin A supplementation may cause harm if supplemented in excess, given the narrow therapeutic window that ongoing alcohol use confers in this cohort. Vitamin A should be supplemented mindfully and on a case-by-case basis. There is a need for further investigation in this area to better elucidate benefits and safety of vitamin A supplementation in patients with ALD.

Vitamin B$_{12}$/Folate

Vitamin B$_{12}$ and folate deficiencies can be seen in patients with chronic alcohol consumption. In hospitalized patients, as many as 80% of patients had folate deficiency and 25% had vitamin B$_{12}$ deficiency.[61] In rat models, treatment with folate and vitamin B$_{12}$ decreases homocysteine levels, which may improve liver injury caused by feeding an ethanol containing diet.[62] The mechanism underlying these deficiencies is complex. Vitamin B$_{12}$ and folate deficiencies are related to the interaction of ethanol and methionine metabolism.[63] Intestinal malabsorption of folate can also occur in chronic alcoholism.[61]

Vitamin B$_{12}$ is vital for the maintenance of myelin function and for hematopoiesis. B$_{12}$ deficiency may cause neurologic complications, including altered mental status and peripheral neuropathy, as well as hematologic complications including macrocytosis, thrombocytopenia, and pancytopenia.[64] Folate deficiency similarly leads to hematologic complications including macrocytic anemia, but does not affect myelin function.[65,66]

Although alcohol itself can cause macrocytosis owing to its direct effects on erythropoiesis resulting in structurally abnormal erythrocytes, macrocytosis in a patient with ALD should trigger an investigation for folate and B$_{12}$ deficiency.[67–69] No consensus recommendations exist regarding scheduled supplementation of B$_{12}$ and folate. When deficiencies in these vitamins exist, they should be treated promptly to avoid the complications discussed herein.[7]

Vitamin D

Vitamin D deficiency is common among patients with chronic liver disease (86.3% in cirrhosis and 49.0% in noncirrhosis),[70] and low bone mineral density can be found in 68% of patients with cirrhosis.[71] Vitamin D deficiency has also been associated with increased liver damage and morality in ALD.[72] The severity of liver disease is a predictor for low vitamin D levels.[73] A single-center, prospective study in Denmark compared effectiveness of a single large dose of ergocalciferol (D$_2$) with cholecalciferol (D$_3$) in patients with alcoholic liver cirrhosis. This study found a supraphysiologic dose of cholecalciferol to be more effective at increasing levels of 25(OH) vitamin D and vitamin D-binding protein measured at days 0, 7, 30, and 90.[74] This study did not include data on the effect on other outcomes such as bone density. Correction of vitamin D deficiency may also improve depressive symptoms in patients with chronic liver disease.[75]

Vitamin E

Vitamin E deficiency may coexist with other fat-soluble vitamin deficiencies. Symptoms of vitamin E deficiency include neurologic deficits, myopathy, and immune cell dysfunction. Vitamin E should not be used as therapy in the absence of deficiency. In animal models of ALD, vitamin E treatment, including the vitamin E analog raxofelast, improves liver histology.[76,77] However, the clinical usefulness of vitamin E in patients with ALD remains questionable. Vitamin E did not improve liver enzymes in patients with mild to moderate alcoholic hepatitis and it did not influence mortality or hospitalization rates in decompensated alcoholic cirrhosis.[78,79]

Zinc

Zinc is important for DNA synthesis, RNA transcription, and cell division. Zinc deficiency can lead to skin lesions, altered taste/smell, encephalopathy, hypogonadism, and altered immune function.[80] Zinc deficiency can be found in approximately 83% of patients with cirrhosis, correlating with disease severity and with decreased transplant-free survival.[81] The underlying mechanism is increased zinc excretion in the urine and decreased absorption in the intestine from alcohol consumption.[56] In 1 small study, zinc supplements administered to patients with alcoholic cirrhosis significantly improved levels of transforming growth factor-β, IL-18, tumor necrosis-α, and Child-Pugh class at 3 months.[36,82] Future high-quality studies are needed to better understand the outcomes, duration and dose of zinc supplementation in ALD.

Patients who suffer from alcoholism can become malnourished through decreased consumption of essential nutrients, postprandial fullness, altered olfaction and gustatory perception, dietary restrictions, alterations in appetite-related hormones, poor absorption, decreased motility, alterations in microbiota, hypermetabolic state, and socioeconomic factors.

SUMMARY

Malnutrition is exceptionally common in patients with ALD, approaching 100% in patients admitted to the hospital for alcoholic hepatitis and in patients with jaundice. Nutritional status should be assessed in patients with ALD, and can be done using simple, inexpensive bedside tests such as the SGA, anthropometry, and handgrip strength. Using serum proteins such as albumin, prealbumin, and transferrin can be misleading owing to decreased synthetic function of the liver and use of intravenous albumin in patients with liver disease. The reasons underlying malnutrition are multifactorial and include caloric intake shifting toward carbohydrates, decreased gastric volume owing to ascites, altered olfactory and gustatory perception, alterations in appetite-related hormones, malabsorption, and potentially altered microbiota. Malnutrition has a significant impact on patient outcomes such as mortality and hospitalization in patients with ALD. Enteral supplementation in both hospital and ambulatory settings may lead to improved outcomes. Additionally, studies continue to emphasize the importance of nutrition in patients with alcoholic hepatitis and patients before and after liver transplantation. Malnutrition has a major impact on the cost of hospitalization for patients with ALD. The mainstays of treatment for malnutrition in ALD include alcohol abstinence and adequate energy and protein intake. Common nutrient deficiencies observed in patients who suffer from ALD include vitamin A, vitamin B_{12}, folate, vitamin D, and zinc. Evaluation for and treatment of such deficiencies is nuanced, and our current understanding of best practices regarding supplementation remains limited.

REFERENCES

1. Soeters P, Bozzetti F, Cynober L, et al. Defining malnutrition: a plea to rethink. Clin Nutr 2017;36(3):896–901.
2. Plauth M, Cabré E, Riggio O, et al. ESPEN guidelines on enteral nutrition: liver disease. Clin Nutr 2006;25(2):285–94.
3. Chao A, Waitzberg D, de Jesus RP, et al. Malnutrition and nutritional support in alcoholic liver disease: a review. Curr Gastroenterol Rep 2016;18(12):65.

4. Campillo B, Richardet JP, Scherman E, et al. Evaluation of nutritional practice in hospitalized cirrhotic patients: results of a prospective study. Nutrition 2003; 19(6):515–21.
5. Marr KJ, Shaheen AA, Lam L, et al. Nutritional status and the performance of multiple bedside tools for nutrition assessment among patients waiting for liver transplantation: a Canadian experience. Clin Nutr ESPEN 2017;17:68–74.
6. Moctezuma-Velázquez C, García-Juárez I, Soto-Solís R, et al. Nutritional assessment and treatment of patients with liver cirrhosis. Nutrition 2013;29(11–12): 1279–85.
7. Rossi RE, Conte D, Massironi S. Diagnosis and treatment of nutritional deficiencies in alcoholic liver disease: overview of available evidence and open issues. Dig Liver Dis 2015;47(10):819–25.
8. Morgan MY, Madden AM, Soulsby CT, et al. Derivation and validation of a new global method for assessing nutritional status in patients with cirrhosis. Hepatology 2006;44(4):823–35.
9. Cheung K, Lee SS, Raman M. Prevalence and mechanisms of malnutrition in patients with advanced liver disease, and nutrition management strategies. Clin Gastroenterol Hepatol 2012;10(2):117–25.
10. Thuluvath PJ, Triger DR. Evaluation of nutritional status by using anthropometry in adults with alcoholic and nonalcoholic liver disease. Am J Clin Nutr 1994;60(2): 269–73.
11. Putadechakum S, Klangjareonchai T, Soponsaritsuk A, et al. Nutritional status assessment in cirrhotic patients after protein supplementation. ISRN Gastroenterol 2012;2012:690402.
12. Pirlich M, Schütz T, Spachos T, et al. Bioelectrical impedance analysis is a useful bedside technique to assess malnutrition in cirrhotic patients with and without ascites. Hepatology 2000;32(6):1208–15.
13. Pirlich M, Selberg O, Böker K, et al. The creatinine approach to estimate skeletal muscle mass in patients with cirrhosis. Hepatology 1996;24(6):1422–7.
14. Brown LA, Cook RT, Jerrells TR, et al. Acute and chronic alcohol abuse modulate immunity. Alcohol Clin Exp Res 2006;30(9):1624–31.
15. O'Keefe SJ, El-Zayadi AR, Carraher TE, et al. Malnutrition and immunoincompetence in patients with liver disease. Lancet 1980;2(8195 pt 1):615–7.
16. Purnak T, Yilmaz Y. Liver disease and malnutrition. Best Pract Res Clin Gastroenterol 2013;27(4):619–29.
17. Alvares-da-Silva MR, Reverbel da Silveira T. Comparison between handgrip strength, subjective global assessment, and prognostic nutritional index in assessing malnutrition and predicting clinical outcome in cirrhotic outpatients. Nutrition 2005;21(2):113–7.
18. Merli M, Giusto M, Gentili F, et al. Nutritional status: its influence on the outcome of patients undergoing liver transplantation. Liver Int 2010;30(2):208–14.
19. Carvalho L, Parise ER. Evaluation of nutritional status of nonhospitalized patients with liver cirrhosis. Arq Gastroenterol 2006;43(4):269–74.
20. Henkel AS, Buchman AL. Nutritional support in patients with chronic liver disease. Nat Clin Pract Gastroenterol Hepatol 2006;3(4):202–9.
21. Huynh DK, Selvanderan SP, Harley HA, et al. Nutritional care in hospitalized patients with chronic liver disease. World J Gastroenterol 2015;21(45):12835–42.
22. Mendenhall C, Roselle GA, Gartside P, et al. Relationship of protein calorie malnutrition to alcoholic liver disease: a reexamination of data from two Veterans Administration Cooperative Studies. Alcohol Clin Exp Res 1995;19(3):635–41.

23. Singal AK, Kamath PS, Francisco Ziller N, et al. Nutritional status of patients with alcoholic cirrhosis undergoing liver transplantation: time trends and impact on survival. Transpl Int 2013;26(8):788–94.

24. Heslin KC, Elixhauser A, Steiner CA. Identifying in-patient costs attributable to the clinical sequelae and comorbidities of alcoholic liver disease in a national hospital database. Addiction 2017;112(5):782–91.

25. Mendenhall CL, Anderson S, Weesner RE, et al. Protein-calorie malnutrition associated with alcoholic hepatitis. Veterans administration cooperative study group on alcoholic hepatitis. Am J Med 1984;76(2):211–22.

26. Lieber CS. Relationships between nutrition, alcohol use, and liver disease. Alcohol Res Health 2003;27(3):220–31.

27. Dasarathy J, McCullough AJ, Dasarathy S. Sarcopenia in alcoholic liver disease: clinical and molecular advances. Alcohol Clin Exp Res 2017;41(8):1419–31.

28. Kumar V, Silvis C, Nystrom G, et al. Alcohol-induced increases in insulin-like growth factor binding protein-1 are partially mediated by TNF. Alcohol Clin Exp Res 2002;26(10):1574–83.

29. Lang CH, Pruznak AM, Deshpande N, et al. Alcohol intoxication impairs phosphorylation of S6K1 and S6 in skeletal muscle independently of ethanol metabolism. Alcohol Clin Exp Res 2004;28(11):1758–67.

30. Thapaliya S, Runkana A, McMullen MR, et al. Alcohol-induced autophagy contributes to loss in skeletal muscle mass. Autophagy 2014;10(4):677–90.

31. Dam G, Sørensen M, Munk OL, et al. Hepatic ethanol elimination kinetics in patients with cirrhosis. Scand J Gastroenterol 2009;44(7):867–71.

32. Dasarathy S. Nutrition and alcoholic liver disease: effects of alcoholism on nutrition, effects of nutrition on alcoholic liver disease, and nutritional therapies for alcoholic liver disease. Clin Liver Dis 2016;20(3):535–50.

33. Aqel BA, Scolapio JS, Dickson RC, et al. Contribution of ascites to impaired gastric function and nutritional intake in patients with cirrhosis and ascites. Clin Gastroenterol Hepatol 2005;3(11):1095–100.

34. Garrett-Laster M, Russell RM, Jacques PF. Impairment of taste and olfaction in patients with cirrhosis: the role of vitamin A. Hum Nutr Clin Nutr 1984;38(3):203–14.

35. Madden AM, Bradbury W, Morgan MY. Taste perception in cirrhosis: its relationship to circulating micronutrients and food preferences. Hepatology 1997;26(1):40–8. Erratum in: Hepatology 1997;26(5):1370.

36. Mohammad MK, Falkner KC, Song M, et al. Low dose zinc sulfate (220mg) supplementation for three months normalizes zinc levels, endotoxemia, pro-inflammatory/fibrotic biomarkers & improves clinical parameters in alcoholic cirrhosis- a double-blind placebo controlled - (ZAC) clinical trial. Hepatology 2015;62:851A.

37. Kalaitzakis E, Bosaeus I, Ohman L, et al. Altered postprandial glucose, insulin, leptin, and ghrelin in liver cirrhosis: correlations with energy intake and resting energy expenditure. Am J Clin Nutr 2007;85(3):808–15.

38. Testa R, Franceschini R, Giannini E, et al. Serum leptin levels in patients with viral chronic hepatitis or liver cirrhosis. J Hepatol 2000;33(1):33–7.

39. Gunnarsdottir SA, Sadik R, Shev S, et al. Small intestinal motility disturbances and bacterial overgrowth in patients with liver cirrhosis and portal hypertension. Am J Gastroenterol 2003;98(6):1362–70.

40. Pace A, de Weerth A, Berna M, et al. Pancreas and liver injury are associated in individuals with increased alcohol consumption. Clin Gastroenterol Hepatol 2009;7(11):1241–6.

41. Ridlon JM, Kang DJ, Hylemon PB, et al. Gut microbiota, cirrhosis, and alcohol regulate bile acid metabolism in the gut. Dig Dis 2015;33(3):338–45.
42. Dasarathy S. Cause and management of muscle wasting in chronic liver disease. Curr Opin Gastroenterol 2016;32(3):159–65.
43. Müller MJ, Lautz HU, Plogmann B, et al. Energy expenditure and substrate oxidation in patients with cirrhosis: the impact of cause, clinical staging and nutritional state. Hepatology 1992;15(5):782–94.
44. Peng S, Plank LD, McCall JL, et al. Body composition, muscle function, and energy expenditure in patients with liver cirrhosis: a comprehensive study. Am J Clin Nutr 2007;85(5):1257–66.
45. Levine JA, Morgan MY. Weighed dietary intakes in patients with chronic liver disease. Nutrition 1996;12(6):430–5.
46. Smith FE, Palmer DL. Alcoholism, infection and altered host defenses: a review of clinical and experimental observations. J Chronic Dis 1976;29(1):35–49.
47. Montano-Loza AJ, Meza-Junco J, Prado CM, et al. Muscle wasting is associated with mortality in patients with cirrhosis. Clin Gastroenterol Hepatol 2012;10(2): 166–73, 173.e1.
48. Huisman EJ, Trip EJ, Siersema PD, et al. Protein energy malnutrition predicts complications in liver cirrhosis. Eur J Gastroenterol Hepatol 2011;23(11):982–9.
49. Hirsch S, Bunout D, de la Maza P, et al. Controlled trial on nutrition supplementation in outpatients with symptomatic alcoholic cirrhosis. JPEN J Parenter Enteral Nutr 1993;17(2):119–24.
50. Fialla AD, Israelsen M, Hamberg O, et al. Nutritional therapy in cirrhosis or alcoholic hepatitis: a systematic review and meta-analysis. Liver Int 2015;35(9):2072–8.
51. Cabré E, Rodríguez-Iglesias P, Caballería J, et al. Short- and long-term outcome of severe alcohol-induced hepatitis treated with steroids or enteral nutrition: a multicenter randomized trial. Hepatology 2000;32(1):36–42.
52. Singal AK, Bataller R, Ahn J, et al. ACG clinical guideline: alcoholic liver disease. Am J Gastroenterol 2018;113(2):175–94.
53. Thursz MR, Forrest EH, Ryder S, STOPAH Investigators. Prednisolone or pentoxifylline for alcoholic hepatitis. N Engl J Med 2015;373(3):282–3.
54. Stephenson GR, Moretti EW, El-Moalem H, et al. Malnutrition in liver transplant patients: preoperative subjective global assessment is predictive of outcome after liver transplantation. Transplantation 2001;72(4):666–70.
55. Hirsch S, de la Maza MP, Gattás V, et al. Nutritional support in alcoholic cirrhotic patients improves host defenses. J Am Coll Nutr 1999;18(5):434–41.
56. Ghorbani Z, Hajizadeh M, Hekmatdoost A. Dietary supplementation in patients with alcoholic liver disease: a review on current evidence. Hepatobiliary Pancreat Dis Int 2016;15(4):348–60.
57. Leo MA, Lieber CS. Hepatic vitamin A depletion in alcoholic liver injury. N Engl J Med 1982;307(10):597–601.
58. Leo MA, Rosman AS, Lieber CS. Differential depletion of carotenoids and tocopherol in liver disease. Hepatology 1993;17(6):977–86.
59. Clugston RD, Blaner WS. The adverse effects of alcohol on vitamin A metabolism. Nutrients 2012;4(5):356–71.
60. Leo MA, Lieber CS. Alcohol, vitamin A, and beta-carotene: adverse interactions, including hepatotoxicity and carcinogenicity. Am J Clin Nutr 1999;69(6):1071–85.
61. Halsted CH, Robles EA, Mezey E. Intestinal malabsorption in folate-deficient alcoholics. Gastroenterology 1973;64(4):526–32.
62. Chen YL, Yang SS, Peng HC, et al. Folate and vitamin B12 improved alcohol-induced hyperhomocysteinemia in rats. Nutrition 2011;27(10):1034–9.

63. Halsted CH. B-Vitamin dependent methionine metabolism and alcoholic liver disease. Clin Chem Lab Med 2013;51(3):457–65.
64. Stabler SP. Vitamin B12 deficiency. N Engl J Med 2013;368(21):2041–2.
65. McClain CJ, Barve SS, Barve A, et al. Alcoholic liver disease and malnutrition. Alcohol Clin Exp Res 2011;35(5):815–20.
66. Medici V, Halsted CH. Folate, alcohol, and liver disease. Mol Nutr Food Res 2013; 57(4):596–606.
67. Wu A, Chanarin I, Levi AJ. Macrocytosis of chronic alcoholism. Lancet 1974; 1(7862):829–31.
68. Morgan MY, Camilo ME, Luck W, et al. Macrocytosis in alcohol-related liver disease: its value for screening. Clin Lab Haematol 1981;3(1):35–44.
69. Ballard HS. The hematological complications of alcoholism. Alcohol Health Res World 1997;21(1):42–52.
70. Fisher L, Fisher A. Vitamin D and parathyroid hormone in outpatients with noncholestatic chronic liver disease. Clin Gastroenterol Hepatol 2007;5(4):513–20.
71. George J, Ganesh HK, Acharya S, et al. Bone mineral density and disorders of mineral metabolism in chronic liver disease. World J Gastroenterol 2009;15(28): 3516–22.
72. Trépo E, Ouziel R, Pradat P, et al. Marked 25-hydroxyvitamin D deficiency is associated with poor prognosis in patients with alcoholic liver disease. J Hepatol 2013;59(2):344–50.
73. Jamil Z, Arif S, Khan A, et al. Vitamin D deficiency and its relationship with Child-Pugh class in patients with chronic liver disease. J Clin Transl Hepatol 2018;6(2): 135–40.
74. Malham M, Peter Jørgensen S, Lauridsen AL, et al. The effect of a single oral megadose of vitamin D provided as either ergocalciferol (D_2) or cholecalciferol (D_3) in alcoholic liver cirrhosis. Eur J Gastroenterol Hepatol 2012;24(2):172–8.
75. Stokes CS, Grünhage F, Baus C, et al. Vitamin D supplementation reduces depressive symptoms in patients with chronic liver disease. Clin Nutr 2016; 35(4):950–7.
76. Hanje AJ, Fortune B, Song M, et al. The use of selected nutrition supplements and complementary and alternative medicine in liver disease. Nutr Clin Pract 2006;21(3):255–72.
77. Nanji AA, Yang EK, Fogt F, et al. Medium chain triglycerides and vitamin E reduce the severity of established experimental alcoholic liver disease. J Pharmacol Exp Ther 1996;277(3):1694–700.
78. Mezey E, Potter JJ, Rennie-Tankersley L, et al. A randomized placebo controlled trial of vitamin E for alcoholic hepatitis. J Hepatol 2004;40(1):40–6.
79. de la Maza MP, Petermann M, Bunout D, et al. Effects of long-term vitamin E supplementation in alcoholic cirrhotics. J Am Coll Nutr 1995;14(2):192–6.
80. Mohammad MK, Zhou Z, Cave M, et al. Zinc and liver disease [review]. Nutr Clin Pract 2012;27(1):8–20. Erratum in: Nutr Clin Pract 2012;27(2):305. Mohommad, Mohammad K [corrected to Mohammad, Mohammad K].
81. Sengupta S, Wroblewski K, Aronsohn A, et al. Screening for zinc deficiency in patients with cirrhosis: when should we start? Dig Dis Sci 2015;60(10):3130–5.
82. Wiegand J, van Bömmel F, Duarte-Rojo A, et al. Clinical trial watch: reports from the liver meeting®, AASLD, San Francisco, November 2015. J Hepatol 2016; 64(6):1428–45.
83. Campillo B, Richardet JP, Bories PN. Validation of body mass index for the diagnosis of malnutrition in patients with liver cirrhosis. Gastroenterol Clin Biol 2006; 30(10):1137–43.

Alcohol-Associated Cirrhosis

Michael R. Lucey, MD

KEYWORDS

• Cirrhosis • Alcohol • Liver disease • Comorbidity

KEY POINTS

- Alcohol-associated cirrhosis (AC) contributes up to 50% of the overall cirrhosis burden in the United States and is likely to become an even greater part of the total burden of liver disease.
- AC is typically a comorbid condition in association with alcohol-use disorder.
- AC is often coexistent with other conditions, both those affecting the liver (hepatitis C virus, hepatitis B virus, hemochromatosis) and others with less obvious connection to the liver (cigarette smoking, hip fractures).

EPIDEMIOLOGY OF ALCOHOL-ASSOCIATED CIRRHOSIS

Alcohol-associated cirrhosis (AC) is thought to contribute up to 50% of the overall cirrhosis burden both in the United States and worldwide.[1] However, as discussed later, in relation to the interrelationship between AC and comorbid disorders, and the phenomenon of clandestine (ie, well-compensated) cirrhosis, the true prevalence of AC is difficult to gauge and likely underestimated.

The histopathologic definitions of cirrhosis and its variants are well described by Nadia Hammoud and Joohi Jimenez-Shahed's article, "Chronic Neurologic Effects of Alcohol," in this issue. This article concentrates on clinical aspects of the presence of cirrhosis in patients with alcohol-use disorder (AUD), and, where possible, on US data, and when discussing regions outside the United States, the country of origin is identified. The prevalence of AC in the United States has been reported in 2 distinct cohorts recently. The prevalence among US veterans has been estimated to be 327 per 100,000,[2] whereas the prevalence rates in a large cohort of privately insured covered lives was approximately 100 per 100,000 enrollees.[3]

Recent studies support 3 broad conclusions with regard to AC in the United States. First, the prevalence of alcohol-related cirrhosis is increasing. Tapper and Parikh[4] studied death certificate data from the Vital Statistics Cooperative and population

Disclosure: The author has nothing to disclose.
Division of Gastroenterology and Hepatology, University of Wisconsin-Madison School of Medicine and Public Health, 1685 Highland Avenue Suite 4000, Madison, WI 53705-2281, USA
E-mail address: mrl@medicine.wisc.edu

liver.theclinics.com

data from the US Census Bureau for the years 1999 to 2016 and found that annual deaths from cirrhosis increased by 65%, whereas annual deaths from hepatocellular carcinoma doubled. Furthermore, data from the most recent interval (2009–2016) showed that persons in the 25-years to 34-years age bracket experienced the highest average annual increase in cirrhosis-related mortality (10.5%, 8.9% to 12.2%, P<.001), driven entirely by alcohol-related liver disease.

The second conclusion is that AC causes disproportionate medical injury and expense compared with other forms of cirrhosis. Mellinger and colleagues[3] used a database of insured persons in 2015, comprising 294,215 persons with cirrhosis, of whom 36% (105,871) were characterized as having AC. When viewed across 7 consecutive years, the AC subcohort were disproportionately sicker at presentation, and readmitted more often, and incurred nearly double the per-person health care costs compared with those with non–alcohol-related cirrhosis.[3]

Third, the proportionate burden of alcohol-related cirrhosis is likely to increase in the next 10 years. Guirguis and colleagues[5] performed a critical overview (rather than a formal meta-analysis) of the existing data and projections for the next decade to assess the likely impact of AC in the next decade. They concluded that, because many of the other causes of cirrhosis are likely to be eclipsed by vaccination (hepatitis B virus) or early effective treatment (hepatitis C virus [HCV]), the contribution of AC to the overall burden of liver disease is likely to increase.

MECHANISMS LEADING TO CIRRHOSIS IN PATIENTS WITH ALCOHOL-USE DISORDER

The mechanisms that underlie the progression to AC have been elegantly described (see Themistoklis Kourkoumpetis and Gagan Sood's article, "Pathogenesis of Alcoholic Liver Disease: An Update," in this issue). The mechanisms described, starting with lipid droplet accumulation within hepatocytes, followed by inflammatory injury, fibrogenesis, and carcinogenesis, all linked to a panel of candidate genetic variants that are key in the pathogenesis of AC, are also key in the progression to HCC, which is discussed briefly later in the article.

INFLUENCE OF COMORBIDITY ON ALCOHOL-ASSOCIATED CIRRHOSIS

Although AUD and alcoholic liver disease (ALD) tend to be described as distinct isolated disorders, they occur in complex interrelations, both with each other and with other disorders. The stigma associated with AUD (see Jessica L. Mellinger and Gerald Scott Winder's article, "Alcohol Use Disorders in Alcoholic Liver Disease," in this issue) has profound importance in the presentation of AC. Because the recognition of the causal role of consumption of alcohol is made through eliciting the patients history, it follows that the role of alcohol may be missed if the patient declines to share this information or is not asked about alcohol-use history. According to data from the United Kingdom, many patients who present for the first time to specialist services with ALD had previously attended their family practitioners with similar symptoms, at which times alcohol use had not been addressed.[6] The emergence of AUD after liver transplant in patients transplanted for other diagnoses is a clear indication of a drinking habit "hiding in plain sight".[7] It follows that the true prevalence of ALD may be underestimated because of a failure of attribution of the primary or coincident cause to excessive alcohol use.

Excessive consumption of alcohol has unwanted synergistic effects on several forms of chronic liver disease, particularly chronic viral hepatitis and metabolic disease, as listed in **Table 1**. The consequences of this interaction include more rapid progression of fibrosis, enhanced risk of development of hepatocellular cancer, and increased rate of death.[8] In recent times, the coincidence of ALD with HCV infection

Table 1
Interaction of alcohol-use disorder and comorbid conditions

Disease	Comment	Reference
Chronic HCV	Promotes cirrhosis at lower doses of alcohol	Corrao & Aricò,[13] 1998
Chronic HBV	In addition to progression, promotes HCC	Ohnishi et al,[14] 1982
NAFLD	Earlier data re benefit in NAFLD of moderate drinking have been refuted	Westin et al,[15] 2002; Naveau et al,[16] 1997
	Alcohol increases the rate of HCC in NASH	Ascha et al,[17] 2010
Hemochromatosis	Excess alcohol increases the expression of cirrhosis	Fletcher et al,[18] 2002
PBC	Moderate drinking linked to fibrosis in 1 study	Sorrentino et al,[19] 2010

Abbreviations: NAFLD, nonalcoholic fatty liver disease; NASH, nonalcoholic steatohepatitis; PBC, primary biliary cirrhosis.

has gained the greatest attention, not least because if its prevalence in at-risk communities.[2] For example, in 2013, out of 5,720,614 patients in US Department of Veterans Affairs care, 60,553 patients (1.06%) had cirrhosis. Among patients with cirrhosis, 35,950 (59%) had AC, comprising 17,546 (29% of the cohort) with combined AC and HCV infection, and 18,404 (30.4%) classified as AC only. However, there are no data to suggest that excessive consumption of alcohol mitigates the effectiveness of direct-acting antiviral agents against HCV.

Patients with AC are at risk for many illnesses and injuries that initially might not seem to be linked to AC. ALD and AC are commonly accompanied by other addictive behaviors, most notably addiction to tobacco. The societal changes in cigarette smoking in the past 50 years are striking, and show that a concerted program of education, combined with consensus-driven changes in social practice, such as increasing the price of cigarettes and creating smoke-free work environments, can effect profound changes. In the United States, adult smoking rates have decreased from ~43% in 1965 to 18% in 2014.[9] Large disparities in tobacco use remain across groups defined by race, ethnicity, educational level, socioeconomic status, and region. In 2014, more than 42 million Americans still smoked on a regular basis, and cigarette smoking remains the chief preventable cause of death in the United States. These data are relevant to the present article because of the high prevalence of cigarette smoking among patients with AC. DiMartini and colleagues[10] have shown that patients with ALD who received liver transplants and who were smokers at the time of their transplants have a high rate of returning to smoking after transplant, and rapidly reach high levels of use. Furthermore, several groups have shown that smoking after transplant has negative impacts on mortality and rates of aerodigestive cancers and cardiovascular disease.[11] It seems reasonable to assume that smoking holds the same risks for patients with AC more generally.

Similarly, recent data from Denmark and the United Kingdom suggest that hip fractures occur more than 5 times more frequently in persons with AC than in people without the disease.[12] In addition, the aftermath of the hip fracture is severe, such that up to 11% of patients with alcoholic cirrhosis die within 30 days after their hip fracture.

MAKING THE DIAGNOSIS OF ALCOHOL-ASSOCIATED CIRRHOSIS

What is the best way to confirm the presence of cirrhosis in an at-risk patient? This question is particularly apposite in patients with AUD who have not experienced a decompensating event such as an episode of jaundice, variceal hemorrhage, encephalopathy, or ascites. Percutaneous liver biopsy is the so-called gold-standard for diagnosis of cirrhosis, but it is invasive, expensive, and carries some risk. Recently, the eclipse of the liver biopsy has been forecast.[20] In its place there is a battery of noninvasive methods, starting with simple blood tests. The circulating platelet count is the most inexpensive surrogate for portal hypertension. **Table 2**, based on the elegant review by Morling and Guha,[21] summarizes the currently available methods, dividing them into liver biopsy, simple indirect markers that are not directly involved in fibrogenesis or lysis (eg, platelet count, aspartate/platelet ratio index, and the Fibrosis-4 index), complex markers that are more directly linked to fibrogenesis and lysis, and measures of liver stiffness in the forms of elastography (shear wave elastography, magnetic resonance elastography).[21,22] In our practice, we use a combination of clinical history and examination, allied with tests: platelet count, elastography, and appearances on trans-sectional imaging. We have a Fibroscan machine (shear wave elastography) in our liver clinic, and encourage patients to come to clinic in a fasted state, thereby permitting serial scans from one clinic visit to the next. It is necessary to be cognizant of the confounding factors, particularly recent drinking, which may increase liver stiffness and thereby mislead the interpreter.[22]

ALCOHOL-ASSOCIATED CIRRHOSIS: NATURAL HISTORY

The natural history of ALD and the sequence of alcoholic steatosis, alcoholic hepatitis (AH), leading to cirrhosis has been described from a histopathologic perspective by Nitzan C. Roth and Jia Qin's article, "Histopathology of Alcohol-Related Liver Diseases," in this issue. Although these distinctions are useful for descriptive purposes, the reality is more complicated. Greater than 50% of patients presenting with a clinical syndrome of AH have established cirrhosis on a contemporaneous biopsy, indicating that the progression to cirrhosis has already begun before the index episode of clinical AH. Furthermore, many patients with AC who have yet to present with a decompensating events (defined as any 1 of the following: variceal hemorrhage, hepatic encephalopathy, jaundice, or ascites) have subtle features of cirrhosis, such as thrombocytopenia or amenorrhea. There are few data on the typical duration of the preclinical phase of AC.

The onset of a decompensating event is a turning point in the natural history of a patient with AC. In 2010, Jepsen and colleagues[23] described the clinical course from the moment of decompensation in a Danish cohort of 466 patients, starting from hospital diagnosis of AC, based on clinical and imaging features with (30%) or without liver biopsy. At diagnosis, 24% were well compensated, 55% had ascites alone, 6% had variceal bleeding alone, 4% had bleeding plus ascites, and 11% had hepatic encephalopathy. During follow-up of a total observation time of 1611 years, 36% of patients maintained abstinent, 43% were intermittent drinkers, and 21% were persistent drinkers. **Fig. 1** shows the clinical course stratified according to the initial presentation. The study provides some important insights. First, most patients at time of hospital diagnosis had already manifested at least 1 decompensating feature. Second, there was no characteristic pattern after presentation and diagnosis. However, the mortality was high across the groups, once they had decompensated. Third, as shown by **Fig. 1**, the decompensating events can occur in concert. The high prevalence of drinking in the cohort no doubt contributed to the outcomes, but the investigators did not analyze outcomes by abstinent versus not abstinent.

Table 2
Comparison of existing and emerging noninvasive markers of hepatic fibrosis

	Liver Biopsy	Indirect Simple Markers	Direct Complex Markers and Cytokines	TE	MR Elastography
Utility in Defining Stage of Fibrosis	Useful for full spectrum	Most useful for advanced fibrosis	Most useful for advanced fibrosis	Most useful for advanced fibrosis	Most useful for advanced fibrosis
Prediction of Clinical Outcomes	HCC, varices	HCC, varices	HCC, varices	HCC, varices	No data presently
Access to and Utility of Serial Assessment	Not practical because of invasive nature	Easily accessible; Emerging data for utility	Easily accessible; Emerging data for utility	Relatively easy access (equipment and experienced operator required); Emerging data for utility	Limited access; No data presently for utility
Financial Costs	$1500 per procedure	Various, $1–$10 per measure	Various, $70–$200 per measure/panel	Capital costs for machine:$60,000; Operational cost: $70 per procedure	Capital costs: >$250,000; Operational cost: $300 per procedure
Reliability	Sampling error (0.00002 of liver sampled)	Laboratory variability	Typically measured at a central laboratory	Operator variability; Reliability reduced in obesity, ascites, liver masses, cholestasis	Limited data available
Performance Location	Hospital	Community or hospital	Community or hospital	Community or hospital	Hospital

Abbreviations: MR, magnetic resonance; TE, transient elastography.
From Morling JR, Guha IN. Biomarkers of liver fibrosis. Clin Liver Dis 2016;7(6):139–42; with permission.

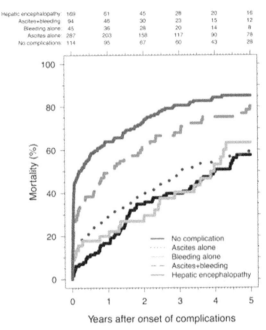

Fig. 1. Clinical course of AC in a Danish population cohort. (*From* Jepsen P, Ott P, Andersen PK, et al. Clinical course of alcoholic liver cirrhosis: a Danish population-based cohort study. Hepatology 2010;51(5):1675–82; with permission.)

THE LINK BETWEEN DRINKING AND DECOMPENSATION

The presentation of and outcome from decompensation are closely linked with drinking. This finding is most obvious in relation to AH, which is defined by the onset of jaundice in close temporal relationship to drinking. Thus, in the context of this article, because 50% or more of patients presenting with AH are cirrhotic, AH can be seen as a decompensating event in cirrhotic patients directly linked to drinking.[24]

Variceal hemorrhage is another informative example, because variceal bleeds often occur after a drinking binge, probably on account of the effect of alcohol on stellate cells in the space of Disse, leading to increased resistance to blood flow in the sinusoids. Even though experiencing AH or hematemesis for the first time is a frightening experience, the complex psychological foundation of addiction is such that the urge to drink still overcomes the fear of hemorrhage and death. This truism is well shown in the Divert Study, which compared portocaval shunt surgery or transjugular intrahepatic portocaval shunts in 140 subjects with a history of at least 1 variceal hemorrhage, about half of whom had AUD (**Fig. 2**).[25] A return to drinking was more common in the patients with AUD, with roughly 25% reporting drinking at each scheduled visit in the course of 60 months' follow-up. Furthermore, a drinking relapse (>4 drinks/d) was recorded in 25 subjects with ALD and no subjects without ALD (*P*<.0001).

As shown in **Fig. 3**, taken from the classic study by Powell and Klatskin,[26] patients who continued to drink after the onset of decompensation experienced a higher mortality than those who were declared abstinent. Although these studies could be criticized for lack of rigor in determining abstinence, they show a clear qualitative difference in the outcome based on drinking. As discussed earlier, AH can be regarded as a decompensating event linked to recent drinking. In recent articles,

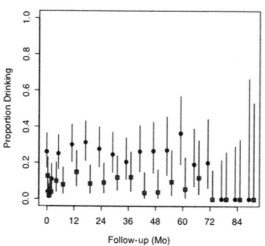

Fig. 2. Proportion of subjects (*blue*, no AUD; *black*, AUD) reporting drinking since their prior visit. (*From* Lucey MR, Connor JT, Boyer TD, et al, DIVERT Study Group. Alcohol consumption by cirrhotic subjects: patterns of use and effects on liver function. Am J Gastroenterol 2008;103(7):1698–706; with permission.)

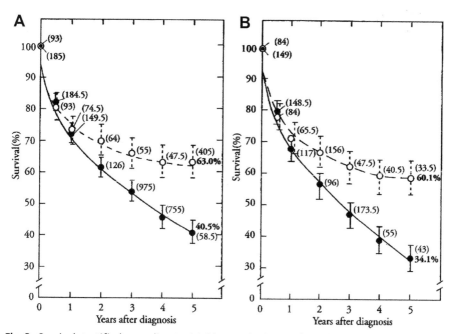

Fig. 3. Survival stratified according to drinking or abstinence from diagnosis of AC (*Panel A*), or first decompensation (*Panel B*). (*From* Powell WJ Jr, Klatskin G. Duration of survival in patients with Laennec's cirrhosis. Influence of alcohol withdrawal, and possible effects of recent changes in general management of the disease. Am J Med 1968;44:406–20; with permission.)

both Louvet and colleagues[27] and Altamirano and colleagues[28] showed in French and Spanish cohorts that long-term survival of patients who recovered from an episode of AH was determined by abstinence.

CAUSE OF DEATH AND ALCOHOL-ASSOCIATED CIRRHOSIS

The outcome of decompensation is stabilization of hepatic function after reestablishing sobriety, or further deterioration and death. In a cohort of 1951 Danish patients with a first-time episode of AH collected between 1999 and 2008, 401 persons died within the first 84 days after admission, and 600 died later.[24] Death in the former group resulted from liver failure (40%), infections (20%), or hepatorenal syndrome (11%). Beyond 84 days, causes of deaths differed between patients with and without cirrhosis; most patients without cirrhosis (n = 326) died of causes related to alcohol abuse, whereas most patients with cirrhosis (n = 675) died of liver failure (34%), infections (16%), or variceal bleeding (11%).

A more particular picture emerges when the events that occur just before death are dissected. Drawing from the example of kidney failure, Moreau and colleagues[29] developed the concept of acute-on-chronic liver failure (ACLF), defined as the clinical status of patients with cirrhosis who have been admitted to hospital with organ failure. ACLF is associated with high mortality. In a landmark article, they used a modified SOFA score, as shown in **Box 1**, to deconstruct 28-day and 90-day mortality in 1343 patients with cirrhosis who were hospitalized. These studies have shown that multisystem organ failure, usually in association with infection, is the process by which cirrhotic patients die. The onset of renal failure is a critical development and the accumulation of failing systems increases the mortality risk.

HEPATOCELLULAR CARCINOMA ARISING IN PATIENTS WITH ALCOHOL-ASSOCIATED CIRRHOSIS

HCC is an additional serious complication of AC that can lead to death. In the Western world, cirrhosis related to both alcohol-associated and non–alcohol-associated steatohepatitis represent common causal pathways for development of HCC. Patients with AC have an estimated risk of developing HCC of 1% to 2% annually.[30] Other factors, including older age, male sex, obesity and diabetes mellitus, and environmental exposure to aflatoxin, represent additional independent predictors for development of HCC in cirrhosis.

Box 1
Elements of the chronic liver failure (CLIF)-sequential organ failure assessment (SOFA) score

1. Liver ~ t bil

2. Kidney ~ serum creatinine

3. Cerebral ~ HE grade

4. Coagulation ~ INR

5. Circulation ~ MAP

6. Respiratory ~ PaO2/FIO2 or SPO2/FIO2

Abbreviations: FIO2, fraction of inspired oxygen; HE, hepatic encephalopathy; INR, International Normalized Ratio; MAP, mean arterial pressure; SPO2, oxygen saturation; t bil, total bilirubin.

MANAGEMENT OF PATIENTS WITH ALCOHOL-ASSOCIATED CIRRHOSIS

All management of AC begins with encouragement to maintain abstinence from alcohol (for a review on the available treatments and barriers to treatment experienced by patients with ALD, see Jessica L. Mellinger and Gerald Scott Winder's article, "Alcohol Use Disorders in Alcoholic Liver Disease," in this issue).

Predicting prognosis in AC is hampered by the confounding effects of drinking. Patients who can achieve stable abstinence have a considerably better prognosis that patients who relapse.[24,27,28] There are no prognostic scoring systems that include continued drinking as a factor. The Model for End-stage Liver Disease (MELD) score (and its more recent iteration including serum sodium [MELD-Na]) offers an indication of 90-day mortality and 1-year mortality.[31] Furthermore, the presence of HCC alters the prognostic predictions.

Patients with AC should receive the same standard of care as patients with other forms of hepatocellular fibrosis and cirrhosis. This care includes interval surveillance for HCC. Current guidelines of the American Association for the Study of Liver Diseases (AASLD) regarding surveillance in patients with cirrhosis advise ultrasonography with or without measurement of alpha fetoprotein every 6 months.[32]

According to the most recent guidelines of the AASLD, patients with AC and accompanying portal hypertension (platelet count <150,000/mm^3) should undergo upper endoscopy to determine the presence of esophagogastric varices.[33] The management of varices is outlined in recent AASLD guidelines.

The management of the other elements of decompensation, such as hepatic encephalopathy and ascites, is also beyond the scope of this article but is codified in societal guidelines (for more information on liver transplantation for ALD, see Elizabeth L. Godfrey and colleagues', "Liver Transplantation for Alcoholic Liver Disease: An Update," in this issue).

PALLIATIVE CARE AND ALCOHOL-ASSOCIATED CIRRHOSIS

Palliative care should be considered for patients with AC who are not candidates for liver transplant, and who are dying, whether because of ACLF, chronic multiorgan failure, or HCC.

Steven Z. Pantilat[34] has described palliative care as "medical care focused on improving quality of life for patients with serious disease." However, the use of palliative care for patients with liver disease, including those with life-limiting AC, has been slow to gain acceptance both with the patient community and among practitioners. In 2014, Poonja and colleagues[35] reported a Canadian retrospective study of 102 consecutive adult patients (67% men; mean age, 55 years) who were removed from the liver transplant list or declined liver transplant from January 2005 through December 2010. Only 11% were referred for palliative care. In the United States, in an analysis of the Nationwide Inpatient Sample, the rate of palliative care referral in end-stage liver disease increased from 0.97% in 2006 to 7.1% in 2012. Referral was influenced by race, insurance status, presence of cancer, do-not-resuscitate status, and being in a large teaching hospital.[36] In my own institution, in a retrospective review of 116 patients declined selection for liver transplant from 2007 to 2012 who subsequently died, 41 patients (35.3%) were referred directly to hospice out of 64 patients (55.2%) who received inpatient or residential hospice care, whereas 32 patients (27.6%) received comfort measures without palliative consultation.[37] Perhaps the most striking observation was that the median survival after palliative care consult or hospice referral was 15 days. Therefore, even in an institution with well-established palliative services, the use of these services occurred very late in each patient's course. The failure to provide palliative care to patients with liver disease with limited expected survival is a missed opportunity. Clinicians have a long way to go to achieve the goal set by Pantilat.[34]

REFERENCES

1. Rehm J, Samokhvalov AV, Shield KD. Global burden of alcoholic liver diseases. J Hepatol 2013;59:160–8.
2. Beste LA, Leipertz SL, Green PK, et al. Trends in burden of cirrhosis and hepatocellular carcinoma by underlying liver disease in US veterans, 2001–2013. Gastroenterology 2015;149:1471–82.e5.
3. Mellinger JL, Shedden K, Winder GS, et al. The high burden of alcoholic cirrhosis in privately insured persons in the United States. Hepatology 2018; 68:872–82.
4. Tapper E, Parikh N. Mortality due to cirrhosis and liver cancer in the United States, 1999-2016: observational study. BMJ 2018;362:k2817.
5. Guirguis J, Chhatwal J, Dasarathy J, et al. Clinical impact of alcohol-related cirrhosis in the next decade: estimates based on current epidemiological trends in the United States. Alcohol Clin Exp Res 2015;39:2085–94.
6. Verrill C, Smith S, Sheron N. Are the opportunities to prevent alcohol related liver deaths in the UK in primary or secondary care? A retrospective clinical review and prospective interview study. Subst Abuse Treat Prev Policy 2006;1:16.
7. Faure S, Herrero A, Jung B, et al. Excessive alcohol consumption after liver transplantation impacts on long-term survival, whatever the primary indication. J Hepatol 2012;57:306–12.
8. Altamirano J, Michelena J. Alcohol consumption as a cofactor for other liver diseases. Clin Liver Dis. Available at: https://aasldpubs.onlinelibrary.wiley.com/doi/10.1002/cld.197.
9. Terry L. The health consequences of smoking: 50 years of progress. A report of the Surgeon General. 2014. Available at: https://www.surgeongeneral.gov/library/reports/50-years-of-progress/index.html.
10. DiMartini A, Javed L, Russell S, et al. Tobacco use following liver transplantation for alcoholic liver disease: an underestimated problem. Liver Transpl 2005;11:679–83.
11. Daniel KE, Eickhoff J, Lucey MR. Why do patients die after a liver transplantation? Clin Transplant 2017;31(3). https://doi.org/10.1111/ctr.12906.
12. Otete H, Deleuran T, Fleming KM, et al. Hip fracture risk in patients with alcoholic cirrhosis: a population-based study using English and Danish data. J Hepatol 2018;69(3):697–704.
13. Corrao G, Aricò S. Independent and combined action of hepatitis C virus infection and alcohol consumption on the risk of symptomatic liver cirrhosis. Hepatology 1998;27:914–9.
14. Ohnishi K, Iida S, Iwama S, et al. The effect of chronic habitual alcohol intake on the development of liver cirrhosis and hepatocellular carcinoma: relation to hepatitis B surface antigen carriage. Cancer 1982;49:672–7.
15. Westin J, Lagging M, Spak F, et al. Moderate alcohol intake increases fibrosis progression in untreated patients with hepatitis C virus infection. J Viral Hepat 2002;9:235–41.
16. Naveau S, Giraud V, Borotto E, et al. Excess weight risk factor for alcoholic liver disease. Hepatology 1997;25:108–11.

17. Ascha MS, Hanouneh IA, Lopez R, et al. The incidence and risk factors of hepatocellular carcinoma in patients with nonalcoholic steatohepatitis. Hepatology 2010;51:1972–8.
18. Fletcher LM, Dixon JL, Purdie DM, et al. Excess alcohol greatly increases the prevalence of cirrhosis in hereditary hemochromatosis. Gastroenterology 2002; 122(2):281–9.
19. Sorrentino P, Terracciano L, D'Angelo S, et al. Oxidative stress and steatosis are cofactors of liver injury in primary biliary cirrhosis. J Gastroenterol 2010;45: 1053–62.
20. Tapper EB, Lok ASF. Use of liver imaging and biopsy in clinical practice. N Engl J Med 2017;377(23):2296–7.
21. Morling JR, Guha IN. Biomarkers of liver fibrosis. Clin Liver Dis 2016. https://doi.org/10.1002/cld.555.
22. Gianni E, Forte P, Galli V, et al. Prospective evaluation of liver stiffness using transient elastography in alcoholic patients following abstinence. Alcohol Alcohol 2017;52(1):42–7.
23. Jepsen P, Ott P, Andersen PK, et al. Clinical course of alcoholic liver cirrhosis: a Danish population-based cohort study. Hepatology 2010;51(5):1675–82.
24. Orntoft NW, Sandahl TD, Jepsen P, et al. Short-term and long-term causes of death in patients with alcoholic hepatitis in Denmark. Clin Gastroenterol Hepatol 2014;12(10):1739–44.e1.
25. Lucey MR, Connor JT, Boyer TD, et al, DIVERT Study Group. Alcohol consumption by cirrhotic subjects: patterns of use and effects on liver function. Am J Gastroenterol 2008;103(7):1698–706.
26. Powell WJ Jr, Klatskin G. Duration of survival in patients with Laennec's cirrhosis. Influence of alcohol withdrawal, and possible effects of recent changes in general management of the disease. Am J Med 1968;44:406–20.
27. Louvet A, Labreuche J, Artru F, et al. Main drivers of outcome differ between short term and long term in severe alcoholic hepatitis: a prospective study. Hepatology 2017;66(5):1464–73.
28. Altamirano J, Lopez-Pelayo H, Michelena J, et al. Alcohol abstinence in patients surviving an episode of alcoholic hepatitis: prediction and long-term impact on survival. Hepatology 2017;66(6):1842–53.
29. Moreau R, Jalan R, Gines P, et al, CANONIC Study Investigators of the EASL–CLIF Consortium. Acute-on-chronic liver failure is a distinct syndrome that develops in patients with acute decompensation of cirrhosis. Gastroenterology 2013;144(7):1426–37, 1437.e1–7.
30. Stickel F. Alcoholic cirrhosis and hepatocellular carcinoma. Adv Exp Med Biol 2015;815:113–30.
31. Said A, Williams J, Holden J, et al. Model for end stage liver disease score predicts mortality across a broad spectrum of liver disease. J Hepatol 2004;40(6): 897–903.
32. Heimbach JK, Kulik LM, Finn RS, et al. AASLD guidelines for the treatment of hepatocellular carcinoma. Hepatology 2018;67(1):358–80. Available at: https://www.aasld.org/sites/default/files/guideline_documents/HCC%20Guideline%202018.pdf.
33. Garcia-Tsao, Abraldes, Berzigotti A, et al. Portal hypertensive bleeding in cirrhosis: risk stratification, diagnosis, and management: 2016 practice guidance by the American Association for the study of liver diseases. Hepatology 2017; 65(1):310–35.
34. Pantilat SZ. Life after the diagnosis. Boston (MA): De Capo Press; 2017.

35. Poonja Z, Brisebois A, van Zanten SV, et al. Patients with cirrhosis and denied liver transplants rarely receive adequate palliative care or appropriate management. Clin Gastroenterol Hepatol 2014;12(4):692–8.
36. Rush B, Walley KR, Celi LA, et al. Palliative care access for hospitalized patients with end-stage liver disease across the United States. Hepatology 2017;66(5): 1585–91.
37. Kelly SG, Campbell TC, Hillman L, et al. The utilization of palliative care services in patients with cirrhosis who have been denied liver transplantation: a single center retrospective review. Ann Hepatol 2017;16(3):395–401.

Liver Transplantation for Alcoholic Liver Disease

An Update

Elizabeth L. Godfrey, BSBE[a],*, Rise Stribling, MD[b],
Abbas Rana, MD[b]

KEYWORDS

- Alcoholic liver disease • Liver transplantation • Alcoholism • End-stage liver disease
- Alcoholic hepatitis

KEY POINTS

- Alcoholic liver disease (ALD) is a prominent contributor to the world liver disease burden. Current research predicts that it is fast becoming the most common cause of end-stage liver disease.
- Determining eligibility for transplantation for ALD requires evaluation of a patient's relapse risk and an effective management plan for the patient's substance use disorders. Integrated alcohol abuse treatment teams should use a mixture of psychosocial and pharmaceutical interventions.
- Patients with ALD require careful management of malnutrition and other comorbidities while on the waitlist. After transplantation, monitoring for de novo malignancy and metabolic conditions is critical.
- Many transplant programs have replaced a mandatory 6-month sobriety period with other requirements because of good outcomes in patients who are transplanted early for severe alcoholic hepatitis.
- Long-term outcomes for transplantation for ALD compare favorably to other indications for liver transplantation. Alcohol relapse occurs in approximately 17% to 22% of patients but only occasionally causes further liver disease.

INTRODUCTION

Alcoholic liver disease (ALD) is a serious contributor to the global liver disease burden, is likely on the increase, and is treatable only with liver transplantation (LT) when sufficiently advanced. Extensive selection criteria, including a specified period of sobriety, has been used in the past to attempt to ensure good outcomes; however, new

Disclosure Statement: The authors have nothing to disclose.
[a] Department of Student Affairs, Baylor College of Medicine, One Baylor Plaza, Houston, TX 77030, USA; [b] 6620 Main Street, Suite 1425, Houston, TX 77030, USA
* Corresponding author.
E-mail address: Elizabeth.Godfrey@bcm.edu

research questions the effectiveness of abstinence periods and has recommended changes in integrated alcohol use treatment to effectively prevent relapse. These patients have unique health concerns, including pretransplantation malnutrition and posttransplantation elevated risk of malignancy, obesity, and cardiac disease. Severe alcoholic hepatitis (AH) has been a condition particularly affected by changing policies surrounding sobriety periods; outcomes of transplanting without a set sobriety period have been favorable, even with respect to rates of recidivism.

EPIDEMIOLOGY OF ALCOHOL USE AND ALCOHOLIC LIVER DISEASE

Alcohol abuse is a global cause of preventable morbidity and mortality. The World Health Organization (WHO) reports that more than 3 million deaths per year are related to harmful alcohol use, accounting for greater than 5% of the global disease burden.[1] It is a disproportionate cause of death in young adults, with far-reaching economic impact; greater than 25% of deaths in the 20 to 39-year-old age group are related to alcohol.[2]

ALD is a spectrum of diseases ranging from fatty liver (a typically reversible effect of heavy alcohol use), to alcoholic cirrhosis, to AH (an acute and severe worsening of liver function). Hepatocellular carcinoma (HCC) may result in the long term. The European Commission reports liver disease as the seventh leading cause of death in Europe, and mortality from liver disease mirrors the pattern of alcohol consumption: where alcohol use is most prevalent, mortality from liver disease is highest.[3,4] In Portugal, where liver disease is the eighth leading cause of death, ALD is the most common form of liver disease and tends to affect younger individuals (typically in their middle age) compared with other forms of liver disease.[4]

Rather than improving with public awareness, ALD rates and mortality have increased over time in the United States. From 2011 to 2013, 81,000 deaths were reported in the United States alone from alcohol-attributable chronic liver disease.[5] American alcohol consumption per capita has been increasing since the 1990s and continues to do so, with a 0.9% increase from 2015 to 2016.[6] A corresponding dramatic increase in cirrhosis mortality has been observed; a 17.5% increase from 2000 to 2015, despite an all-cause mortality decline of 15.6%.[7] Alcohol is projected to become the single most common cause of cirrhosis in the United States in the next decade, replacing hepatitis C virus (HCV) and other viral causes.[8]

ALD has long been known to be a major cause of morbidity and mortality in Europe and North America; however, emerging research in Latin America and Asia indicates its increasingly global impact. Although nonalcoholic fatty liver disease has received considerable attention in recent years, ALD continues to be either a stable or increasing cause of HCC and related orthotopic LT (OLT) in Latin America.[9] Moreover, some of the fastest rates of increase of ALD have been reported in countries such as China and India. Given their large populations and disparities in health care surveillance and reporting, ALD will likely remain an underreported source of morbidity and mortality, particularly in low-reporting areas.[10,11]

Additionally, alcohol consumption in several countries worldwide continues to increase, often in the younger population and in women, in Europe as well in nations such as Korea.[2,12] In the coming years, as those individuals age, this is likely to prefigure an even more dramatic increase in ALD despite a recent drop in older individuals presenting with ALD.[12]

LIVER TRANSPLANTATION AND ALCOHOLIC LIVER DISEASE

ALD is the major indication for LT worldwide. In the United States and Europe, it was the second most common indication for transplant, behind chronic HCV, before 2016.[13]

Since then, ALD has become and is projected to remain the single largest known indication for OLT in the United States.[8,14] The percentage of liver transplants attributed to alcoholic cirrhosis has increased from 12.8% in 2002 to 16.5% in 2010.[8,14,15]

This epidemiologic shift in the indication for listing for transplant is due in large part to decreased incidence of HCV cirrhosis.[14] Given the meteoric increase in obesity and fatty liver disease, one might expect nonalcoholic steatohepatitis (NASH)-related cirrhosis to become the number 1 indication for OLT. NASH-related cirrhosis is actually the second most common reason for a patient's addition to the OLT waitlist; however, many hope that promising drugs in development will reduce the number of patients for whom OLT is the destination therapy of choice.[16]

The only effective treatments for severe ALD are alcohol abstinence and transplantation.[16] Many pharmaceuticals agents have been studied in this population, several of which have been widely prescribed, only to be called into question after further study. Propylthiouracil, colchicine, s-adenosyl-L-methionine, and polyenylphosphatidylcholine are some agents that are now considered of marginal value.[17] Propylthiouracil is the only therapy accepted on meta-analysis to have some evidence to support its use for ALD; however, it has not been studied for many years and is clearly ineffective for acute AH.[17] Despite a lack of treatment options, many ALD patients are never listed for transplantation, although those with concomitant HCC are much more likely to be listed.[18] There are experimental therapies for use in ALD. (See Vinay Sundaram and Timothy R. Morgan's article, "Will Studies in Nonalcoholic Steatohepatitis Help Manage Alcoholic Steatohepatitis?," in this issue.)

ALCOHOLIC LIVER DISEASE IN THE PRETRANSPLANT PERIOD

Patients with end-stage ALD present several clinical challenges in the pretransplant period. They suffer from a wide variety of comorbidities, including sarcopenia, neurologic disorders, kidney dysfunction (including acute kidney injury, particularly in AH), cardiovascular disease, and psychological comorbidities, especially depression.[19,20] Nearly all ALD patients are also to some extent malnourished, particularly in terms of protein-energy malnutrition, micronutrients such as zinc, and vitamins such as thiamine. All these require monitoring and supplementation.[19,21]

Indications and contraindications for LT in patients with end-stage ALD are similar to those for other causes; however, there is an additional focus on selecting patients who are less likely to relapse into harmful alcohol use.[13] Before referring a patient with end-stage liver disease for transplantation, even if their primary disease is not ALD, a detailed history of the patient's alcohol and other substance use, and their consequences, is required. The preferred simple, standardized questionnaire to screen for excessive alcohol use in any patient is the WHO Alcohol Use Disorders Identification Test (AUDIT); a free version is available from National Institute on Alcohol Abuse and Alcoholism (NIAAA) Web site (http://pubs.niaaa.nih.gov/publications/Audit.pdf).[13,22]

Typically, ALD patients are expected to demonstrate abstinence from alcohol for a specified time before listing. The current 6-month rule dates back to 1997, when a consensus document from American LT physicians recommended 6 months of abstinence before listing.[23,24] Over time, these guidelines have been questioned, particularly for acutely ill patients. A variety of European and, later, American studies over the past decade demonstrated multiple successful series of early transplantation for severe AH (sAH), with recidivism rates comparable with or lower than ALD cohorts who completed a period of alcohol abstinence before listing.[25-27]

European institutions were the first to change their recommendations: consensus conferences since 2006 in the United Kingdom and France did not recommend a fixed abstinence period.[28,29] The International Liver Transplant Society's most recent recommendations continue to recommend some period of abstinence, with 6 months likely to remain a common benchmark, but also recommends evaluating patients for transplant if medical urgency precludes the traditional waiting period.[30] Additionally, the American Gastroenterological Association (AGA) Institute now recommends referral for transplantation for sAH for patients with good social support and acceptable insight, and has removed the minimum sobriety period.[31]

Although requirements are now more flexible, a period of abstinence still has considerable utility. It identifies patients who will recover hepatic function and it helps exclude those individuals who cannot abstain from drinking.[32,33] The problem with specifying any particular time period is that only much longer periods of abstinence are likely to be effective in determining recidivism. A study in Japan indicated that 18 months may be effective.[34] A US database study correlated 2 years or more of pre-LT abstinence with less post-LT alcohol use, and a scoring system study found that relapsers had had an average of 27.7 months of abstinence.[35,36] Such long periods of abstinence are not practical given the rapid disease course of some patients. Other methods of reducing recidivism are necessary.

Beyond abstinence periods, assessing and reducing the risk of posttransplant harmful drinking is key. Recidivism is widespread: approximately a quarter of LT recipients, whether they were listed for ALD or some other cause, report relapse of alcohol use.[35,36] Currently, objective risk assessment remains elusive; no single instrument precisely estimates risk of relapse after liver transplant.[13]

Several positive and negative factors associated with recidivism have been identified. Favorable outcomes are associated with the patient's acknowledgment of addiction, age older than 40 years; an ample social support system (particularly a spouse), a job, a home, social integration, activities to replace drinking in daily life, support of rehabilitation relationship, source of improved self-esteem or of hope for the future, and identification by the patient of the negative consequences of returning to drinking.[37] Cigarette smoking and psychiatric comorbidities, conversely, are associated with return to drinking.[37,38] Although a 6-month period of abstinence does not effectively reduce recidivism, a short duration of sobriety (<6 months) may be a significant predictor of time to first drink and time to bingeing.[38] A positive family history of alcoholism can also indicate individuals more likely to return to drinking.[13,39]

Although no single instrument fully estimates relapse risk, a few scoring systems may be useful. One example is the Stanford Integrated Psychosocial Assessment for Transplantation (SIPAT), which uses 18 risk factors in the 4 domains of patient readiness, social support, psychological stability, and substance abuse. Its strengths include standardization of the evaluation process and its ability to identify those at risk for negative outcomes. The SIPAT has been validated in liver, lung, kidney, and heart recipients to predict "secondary medical and psychosocial outcomes such as rejection episodes, hospitalizations, infections and psychosocial decompensation."[37,40,41] The High-Risk Alcohol Relapse (HRAR) inventory is another potentially useful instrument. It assesses duration of heavy drinking, number of drinks per day, and number of prior alcoholism inpatient treatment experiences with a simple 3-by-3 scale. It was not validated in some studies; however, in others, the HRAR was found to be highly predictive of relapse. A score greater than 3 predicted relapse with an odds ratio of 10.7 (P = .001).[37,38,42] The Alcohol Relapse Risk Assessment (ARRA) score has also shown promise. Using 9 independent factors, it predicted moderate and heavy relapse with an area under the curve (AUC) of 0.892. However, it has had fairly limited validation to date and needs further study.[36,37]

After a patient's eligibility has been determined, he or she must be monitored for potential relapse while on the waitlist. The first-line monitoring method is to directly ask the patient and his or her support system about relapse. The reliability of thorough interviewing of the patient and family has been formally demonstrated through research into alcohol relapse. One Australian study showed that married subjects are more likely to be reported for relapse than unmarried subjects. This most likely reflects better insight and assessment by the spouse rather than a higher prevalence of drinking among married people.[43]

Some laboratory tests may provide useful supplemental methods. Current recommended and widely available alcohol use monitoring techniques include blood testing for gamma glutamyl transferase (GGT) and carbohydrate-deficient transferrin. Other direct markers include blood ethanol, methanol, ethyl sulfate, phosphatidyl ethanol, and urine ethyl glucuronide.[44] Unfortunately, GGT, although relatively available, is very specific with low sensitivity and can easily fail to detect a patient's relapse.[45] Urine ethyl glucuronide is very sensitive and effective within up to 4 to 5 days of alcohol consumption but requires frequent testing and is known to generate false positives.[44,45] Carbohydrate-deficient transferrin accurately assesses alcohol consumption in the general population but is less accurate in patients with cirrhosis, women, and the obese, which collectively accounts for most individuals with ALD.[46]

If a waitlisted patient does relapse, he or she should receive further dependency counseling and should be made inactive on the list or delisted until abstinence is achieved and sustained.[47] Programs with in-house counseling and dependency services, most notably when cognitive behavioral and medical treatments are provided together, have shown enhanced effectiveness in inducing and maintaining alcohol abstinence.[48] Multidisciplinary teams are crucial to managing these patients at all stages of care. To increase success, a multidisciplinary team evaluation must be conducted initially to develop a treatment plan for the patient's liver disease, to assess a patient's transplant candidacy, and to establish a management plan for the patient's alcoholism.[13]

POSTTRANSPLANT OUTCOMES IN ALCOHOLIC LIVER DISEASE

Posttransplant outcomes for alcoholic cirrhosis have been good when compared with other indications for transplantation. Post-LT survival rates at 1, 3, 5, and 10 years are reported to be between 84% and 89%, 78% and 83%, 73% and 79%, and 58% and 73%, respectively. These are higher than rates reported for HCV cirrhosis or HCC, and similar to other indications for transplant.[49,50] However, in individuals who do not remain alcohol-abstinent, outcomes are poorer and death from liver-related causes is higher than in viral or non-ALD.[51]

In relapsing patients, 10-year survival is significantly lower, between 45% and 71% compared with 75% and 93% among abstinent patients or those with only occasional slips.[52–55] Emerging data further describe a greater incidence of progressive liver injury and additional episodes of AH and cirrhosis in relapsing patients.[53,56–58] Unfortunately, this also affects a substantial number of patients. Recent studies estimate clinically significant relapse rates between 18% and 50% of recipients transplanted for ALD, although varied definitions of relapse make this difficult to assess.[55,59]

One prospective study at the University of Pittsburgh monitored alcohol use for more than 10 years and found that early relapse was the most harmful single behavior. By 10 years, about 50% of recipients had consumed some alcohol.[60] Moderate or heavy users who resumed alcohol early after transplant were more likely to exhibit rejection or steatohepatitis on biopsy and more likely to progress to graft failure than recipients who waited longer to resume alcohol use, even if their consumption was heavier. Furthermore, all individuals who experienced recurrent liver disease were in the early-relapse groups. Factors that contributed to relapse included family history and short sobriety periods before OLT.[60]

In a prospective study at the University of Wisconsin, relapsed subjects experienced a 3-fold increased rate of graft loss compared with abstainers. Subjects who returned to drinking were more likely to have steatosis, steatohepatitis, and advanced fibrosis at or higher than stage 3.[57] This study also refuted the conjecture that relapsed patients have decreased adherence to immunosuppressive drugs: ductopenia was not observed.[57] Several other studies have also suggested that there is minimal difference in rejection between relapsed and nonrelapsed subjects.[53]

Finally, a retrospective study of 712 subjects, among the largest studies on long-term post-LT outcomes, reported severe relapse in 128 subjects, or approximately 18%. Such relapses led to recurrent alcoholic cirrhosis in 32% of individuals, with significantly decreased long-term survival. The study demonstrated 1-year, 5-year, 10-year, and 15-year subject survival rates of 100%, 88%, 50%, and 21%, respectively, for cases of recurrent alcoholic cirrhosis, and of 100%, 89%, 70%, and 41%, for subjects without recurrence (P<.001). Individuals who relapse have similar liver disease recurrence rates as HCV cirrhosis patients.[59]

In conclusion, ALD patients are likely to have excellent outcomes as long as alcohol abstinence is maintained.

CONSIDERATIONS FOR POSTTRANSPLANTATION CARE

Posttransplantation care involves a variety of disease-specific monitoring and preventative health care interventions in addition to continued recidivism awareness. Patients with LT due to ALD should be screened regularly for HCC and other gastrointestinal cancers because their risk of de novo malignancy is 2 or 3 times higher than controls, and even more so in individuals who resume drinking.[49,59] Smoking, which is common in this population, further increases risk of de novo malignancy, including intrahepatic and extrahepatic cholangiocarcinoma.[61] Patients should be persistently encouraged to participate in smoking cessation treatment.

Obesity remains a problem affecting most patients but is particularly concerning in the post-OLT population. Elevated body mass index is associated with increased risk of cirrhosis, and may exacerbate diabetes, hypertension, and cardiovascular sequelae, which are commonly found in post-OLT patients.[62,63] Type 2 diabetes, if it develops, is associated with a 40-fold higher cancer risk in patients with a history of ALD.[64] Patients should be reminded that obesity is the most insidious threat to the success of their liver transplant.

Monitoring for resumption of harmful alcohol consumption remains key in post-transplant management. A variety of therapies and methodologies have been studied for preventing recidivism. Recent data supports in-house counseling teams and combined psychosocial and medical therapy. One Italian program studied recidivism before and after implementation of an alcohol addiction unit, an interdisciplinary program including internists and psychologists, with mixed expertise in alcoholism, hepatology, and neuroscience. This integrated counseling team, which was in-house but not directly connected to the institution's transplantation program, had a positive protective effect against recidivism (odds ratio [OR] 0.23) and death (OR 0.28).[65] Although this study suffered from several limitations, other studies have generated similar conclusions. In-house teams that are not actively part of the transplant team (and therefore not responsible for any changes in care that could be perceived as punitive, which often affects patients' willingness to seek care) may be the most likely to obtain honest, actionable responses from patients about their alcohol use.[66,67]

It has been suggested that alcohol abuse treatment after transplant may be more critical than before transplant. One study showed improved outcomes were associated with alcohol abuse treatment after transplant, whereas treatment before was not significantly better than no treatment.[68] This study also evaluated treatment intensity, which was not found to significantly affect outcomes. One caveat of this finding is that more ill patients are less able to engage in higher intensity treatment. Another potential limitation of this conclusion is that the subjects were not randomized to different intensities of treatment or treatment periods; subjects considered to have more severe alcohol use disorders may have been the ones receiving the most extensive therapy.[68] After-transplant therapy is still nevertheless implicated as a meaningful step in maintaining alcohol abstinence.

A combination of psychosocial and medical therapy may be the most effective approach in this population. A systematic review concluded, based on several recent research studies, that psychosocial therapies alone are not effective in improving outcomes.[48] Specifically, a combination of cognitive behavioral, motivational enhancement, and medical therapy was shown overall to be the only method fully supported by the data.[48] Again, substance abuse therapy in this context may have the best performance when administered by integrated treatment teams.[69]

LIVER TRANSPLANTATION IN ALCOHOLIC HEPATITIS

Much of the recent research regarding LT in ALD has been dedicated to AH, with increasing focus on LT in sAH. Because sAH is typically too acute to permit a period of alcohol abstinence, determining appropriate selection protocols and recidivism prevention methods has been crucial in this population.

AH is a distinct syndrome seen in patients with chronic alcohol use. It is characterized by worsening jaundice and elevated serum aspartate transaminase (>50 IU/mL). The NIAAA specifies the following diagnostic criteria: "Serum bilirubin is usually elevated (>3 mg/dL [>50 μmol/L]), as is the AST (>50 IU/mL), and AST [aspartate transaminase] to alanine aminotransferase (ALT) ratio of >1.5."[70]

AH causes significant morbidity and mortality in the short-term compared with chronic ALD, with mortality of 25% at 28 days and 44% at 180 days.[71] Moreover, mortality rates have not improved over time; in fact, mortality at 180 days after admission has shown a statistically significant increase since the 1970s.[71] Most individuals with sAH also have cirrhosis and most will have alcoholic steatotic hepatitis on biopsy.[70] Additionally, AH has a high association with infection, particularly nosocomial infections in the setting of steroid therapy.[72]

Limited treatment options are available for AH outside of transplantation. Prednisone and pentoxifylline have been recommended in the past; however, their benefits were questioned by a UK randomized controlled trial that showed no 28-day, 90-day, or 1-year survival advantage, and reported increased infection rates in prednisolone recipients.[73] Of note, prednisolone did not increase infections during therapy but did afterward. If infected, subjects also exhibited elevated 90-day mortality.[74] Another large retrospective study even indicated numerically increased (though statistically nonsignificant) mortality in the treatment group, perhaps because sAH is already too far progressed to be improved by pharmaceutical methods.[20] It has been conjectured that pentoxifylline may have therapeutic benefit but only in patients with hepatorenal syndrome.[75] Overall, because there are no better options, the AGA and others continue to recommend treatment with pentoxifylline based on the studies that showed some benefit.[31]

With so few options for treatment, it became clear over the past several years that transplantation protocols would have to change to address this population's need. If long sobriety periods were required for transplantation, then these patients would have no options left open to them. French consensus recommendations were the earliest to abandon a specific length of sobriety; an early multicenter prospective trial of OLT for sAH was reported in 2011.[27] Unsurprisingly, 6-month survival was vastly higher in subjects who received early OLT (77% vs 23%), and that benefit persisted over 2 years of follow-up. Only 3 of the 26 relapsed.[27]

Building on promising studies such as this from Europe, a study of 80 US transplant recipients (34 with cirrhosis and 46 with sAH) was conducted, waiving the 6-month abstinence rule for the sAH recipients. Harmful drinking patterns were resumed over the course of follow-up in 12% and 17% of each group, respectively (a nonsignificant difference). Subjects with sAH had outcomes similar to any transplant for ALD, with no difference in 6-month or 1-year recipient or graft survival. When adjusted for age and social factors as measured by Hopkins Psychosocial Scale, subjects with sAH were not more likely to relapse.[26]

The largest retrospective study to date, studying 147 liver recipients from 12 US centers transplanted for sAH, has recently gone to press. Subjects' 1-year survival and 3-year survival were excellent at 94% and 84%, respectively, which is higher than HCC and, in fact, most indications for LT. Cumulative probability of any alcohol use at 1 and 3 years was 25% and 34%, respectively; however, more than half of those instances were isolated slips and only 11% of individuals returned to sustained drinking patterns. One limitation of this study, however, was that many subjects met clinical but not histologic AH requirements.[76] Nevertheless, transplantation for sAH boasts good outcomes. A meta-analysis of existing sAH studies suggests relapse rates of 0.22, which are at least equivalent if not favorable in comparison with other ALD-indicated transplantation.[25]

One concern about continuing to increase transplantation in this population has been fear of negative public opinion, particularly concerns that such policies could reduce public willingness to donate organs. A review of survey studies suggests there is some foundation to these concerns: the public, and to a lesser extent physicians, are relatively biased against transplant for ALD compared with conditions that are not related to patient behavior. However, despite occasional public outcry against such donation practices, the actual number of organ donors has not changed.[77] A US-based marketplace survey in 2015 measured attitudes about LT for ALD and early transplant for AH. Only a minority of respondents were unwilling to use organs on patients with alcohol-induced disease. Respondents rated the age of the prospective recipient as the most important selection factor and financial stability the least, and viewed middle-aged patients with good social support most favorably. This suggests that public opinion is more in line with early transplant for sAH than had previously been suspected.[78]

SUMMARY

ALD, a major cause of global morbidity and mortality, is likely to continue to increase in the global health burden over the coming years. Although several new therapies have become available for other causes of liver disease, very few effective therapies exist for ALD other than LT. To ensure good outcomes and appropriate allocation of scarce donated organs, stringent selection criteria must be used to determine who is eligible to receive a graft, and effective, integrated alcohol use treatment must be used to prevent relapse. In addition to assiduous monitoring for alcohol use relapse before and after transplantation, these patients must also be managed for their unique health concerns, including pretransplantation malnutrition and posttransplantation elevated risk of malignancy, obesity, and cardiac disease. Older transplantation practices limited transplants to those patients who were able to demonstrate 6 months of sobriety; however, more flexible guidelines are emerging to address those with more acute conditions such as sAH. Outcomes have been good, supporting continued flexibility in selection and treatment protocols.

REFERENCES

1. WHO. Global status report on alcohol and health. World Heal Organ; 2014. p. 1–100. Available at: https://doi.org//entity/substance_abuse/publications/global_alcohol_report/en/index.html.
2. Pimpin L, Cortez-pinto H, Negro F, et al. Burden of liver disease in Europe : epidemiology and analysis of risk factors to identify prevention policies. J Hepatol 2018;69(3):718–35.
3. European Commission. Eurostats pocketbooks: European social statistics–2013 edition. Luxembourg: Publications Office of the European Union; 2013.
4. Coelho M, Marinho RT, Rodrigues T. Mortality associated with hepatobiliary disease in Portugal between 2006 and 2012. GE Port J Gastroenterol 2018;25:123–31.
5. Tomedi LE, Roeber J, Landen M. Alcohol consumption and chronic liver disease mortality in New Mexico and the United States, 1999-2013. Public Health Rep 2018;133(3):287–93.
6. Haughwout SP, Slater ME. Apparent per capita alcohol consumption: national, state, and regional trends, 1977–2016. Arlington (VA): 2016. Available at: https://pubs.niaaa.nih.gov/publications/surveillance104/CONS14.htm. Accessed May 29, 2019.
7. Yoon YH, Chen CM. Liver cirrhosis mortality in the United States: national, state, and regional trends, 2000-2015 (surveillance report #111). Arlington (VA): 2016. Available at: https://pubs.niaaa.nih.gov/publications/surveillance105/Cirr13.pdf. Accessed May 29, 2019.
8. Guirguis J, Chhatwal J, Dasarathy J, et al. Clinical impact of alcohol-related cirrhosis in the next decade: estimates based on current epidemiological trends in the United States. Alcohol Clin Exp Res 2015;39(11):2085–94.
9. Piñero F, Costa P, Boteon YL, et al. Results of liver transplantation for hepatocellular carcinoma in a multicenter Latin American cohort study. Ann Hepatol 2018; 17(2):8–10.
10. Tang YL, Xiang XJ, Wang XY, et al. L'alcool et ses méfaits en Chine: les changements politiques nécessaires. Bull World Health Organ 2013;91(4):270–6.
11. Liangpunsakul S, Haber P, McCaughan GW. Alcoholic liver disease in Asia, Europe, and North America. Gastroenterology 2016;150(8):1786–97.
12. Jang JY, Kim DJ. Epidemiology of alcoholic liver disease in Korea. Clin Mol Hepatol 2018;8:12–25.
13. Gallegos-Orozco JF, Charlton MR. Alcoholic liver disease and liver transplantation. Clin Liver Dis 2016;20(3):521–34.
14. Kim WR, Lake JR, Smith JM, et al. OPTN/SRTR 2016 annual data report. Liver 2016. https://doi.org/10.1111/ajt.14560.
15. Kling CE, Perkins JD, Carithers RL, et al. Recent trends in liver transplantation for alcoholic liver disease in the United States. World J Hepatol 2017;9(36):1315–21.

16. Goldberg D, Ditah IC, Saeian K, et al. Changes in the prevalence of hepatitis C virus infection, nonalcoholic steatohepatitis, and alcoholic liver disease among patients with cirrhosis or liver failure on the waitlist for liver transplantation. Gastroenterology 2017;152(5):1090–9.e1.

17. Elena B, Maria K, Douglas T, et al. Pharmacological interventions for alcoholic liver disease (alcohol-related liver disease). 2017;3. https://doi.org/10.1002/14651858.CD011646.pub2. Available at: www.cochranelibrary.com. Accessed May 29, 2019.

18. Goldberg D, French B, Newcomb C, et al. Patients with hepatocellular carcinoma have highest rates of wait-listing for liver transplantation among patients with end-stage liver disease. Clin Gastroenterol Hepatol 2016;14(11):1638–46.e2.

19. Stickel F, Datz C, Hampe J, et al. Pathophysiology and management of alcoholic liver disease: update 2016. Gut Liver 2017;11(2):173–88.

20. Owens RE, Snyder HS, Twilla JD, et al. Pharmacologic treatment of alcoholic hepatitis: examining outcomes based on disease severity stratification. J Clin Exp Hepatol 2016;6(4):275–81.

21. Kharbanda KK, Ronis MJJ, Shearn CT, et al. Role of nutrition in alcoholic liver disease: summary of the symposium at the ESBRA 2017 congress. Biomolecules 2018;8(2). https://doi.org/10.3390/biom8020015.

22. Babor T. AUDIT: the alcohol use disorders identification test. In: National Institute on Alcohol and Alcoholism, editor. Helping patients who drink too much: A clinician's guide. Bethesda: National Institutes of Health. p. 1–40. NIH publication No. 07-3769. Available at: https://pubs.niaaa.nih.gov/publications/Audit.pdf.

23. Hoofnagle JH, Kresina T, Fuller RK, et al. Liver transplantation for alcoholic liver disease: executive statement and recommendations. Clin Liver Dis 2013;2(2):92–5. Available at: http://www.embase.com/search/results?subaction=view record&from=export&id=L368821552%5Cnhttps://doi.org/10.1002/cld.204%5Cnhttp://mgetit.lib.umich.edu/sfx_locater?sid=EMBASE&issn=20462484&id=doi:10.1002%2Fcld.204&atitle=Liver+transplantation+for+alcoholi.

24. Lucey MR. Issues in selection for and outcome of liver transplantation in patients with alcoholic liver disease. Liver Transpl Surg 1997;3(3):227–30.

25. Marot A, Dubois M, Trépo E, et al. Liver transplantation for alcoholic hepatitis: a systematic review with meta-analysis. PLoS One 2018;13(1):1–14.

26. Weeks SR, Sun Z, McCaul ME, et al. Liver transplantation for severe alcoholic hepatitis, updated lessons from the world's largest series. J Am Coll Surg 2018;226(4):549–57.

27. Mathurin P, Moreno C, Samuel D, et al. Early liver transplantation for severe alcoholic hepatitis. N Engl J Med 2011;365:1790–800.

28. Bathgate A. Recommendations for alcohol-related liver disease. Lancet 2006;367(9528):2045–6.

29. Webb K, Shepherd L, Day E, et al. Transplantation for alcoholic liver disease: report of a consensus meeting. Liver Transpl 2006;12(2):301–5.

30. Addolorato G, Bataller R, Burra P, et al. Liver transplantation for alcoholic liver disease. Transplantation 2016;100(5):981–7.

31. Mitchell MC, Friedman LS, McClain CJ. Medical management of severe alcoholic hepatitis: expert review from the clinical practice updates committee of the AGA institute. Clin Gastroenterol Hepatol 2017;15(1):5–12.

32. Hagström H. Alcohol, smoking and the liver disease patient. Best Pract Res Clin Gastroenterol 2017;31(5):537–43.

33. Kubiliun M, Patel SJ, Hur C, et al. Early liver transplantation for alcoholic hepatitis: ready for primetime? J Hepatol 2018;68(3):380–2.

34. Egawa H, Ueda Y, Kawagishi N, et al. Significance of pretransplant abstinence on harmful alcohol relapse after liver transplantation for alcoholic cirrhosis in Japan. Hepatol Res 2014;44(14):E428–36.
35. Russ KB, Chen NW, Kamath PS, et al. Alcohol use after liver transplantation is independent of liver disease etiology. Alcohol Alcohol 2016;51(6):698–701.
36. Rodrigue J, Hanto D, Curry M. The Alcohol Relapse Risk Assessment: a scoring system to predict the risk of relapse to any alcohol use after liver transplant. Prog Transplant 2013;23(4):310–8.
37. Lim J, Curry MP, Sundaram V. Risk factors and outcomes associated with alcohol relapse after liver transplantation. World J Hepatol 2017;9(17):771–80.
38. De Gottardi A, Spahr L, Gelez P, et al. A simple score for predicting alcohol relapse after liver transplantation. Arch Intern Med 2007;167(11):1183.
39. Dew MA, DiMartini AF, Steel J, et al. Meta-analysis of risk for relapse to substance use after transplantation of the liver or other solid organs. Liver Transpl 2008; 14(2):159–72.
40. Maldonado JR, Dubois HC, David EE, et al. The Stanford Integrated Psychosocial Assessment for Transplantation (SIPAT): a new tool for the psychosocial evaluation of pre-transplant candidates. Psychosomatics 2012;53(2):123–32.
41. Maldonado JR, Sher Y, Lolak S, et al. The Stanford integrated psychosocial assessment for transplantation: a prospective study of medical and psychosocial outcomes. Psychosom Med 2015;77(9):1018–30.
42. Altamirano J, López-Pelayo H, Michelena J, et al. Alcohol abstinence in patients surviving an episode of alcoholic hepatitis: prediction and impact on long-term survival. Hepatology 2017;66(6):1842–53.
43. Wigg AJ, Mangira D, Chen JW, et al. Outcomes and predictors of harmful relapse following liver transplantation for alcoholic liver disease in an Australian population. Intern Med J 2017;47(6):656–63.
44. Allen JP, Wurst FM, Thon N, et al. Assessing the drinking status of liver transplant patients with alcoholic liver disease. Liver Transpl 2013;19(4):369–76.
45. Whitfield JB, Masson S, Liangpunsakul S, et al. Evaluation of laboratory tests for cirrhosis and for alcohol use, in the context of alcoholic cirrhosis. Alcohol 2018; 66:1–7.
46. Fagan KJ, Irvine KM, McWhinney BC, et al. Diagnostic sensitivity of carbohydrate deficient transferrin in heavy drinkers. BMC Gastroenterol 2014;14(1):1–6.
47. Sterneck M, Yegles M, Rothkirch von G, et al. Determination of ethyl glucuronide in hair improves evaluation of long-term alcohol abstention in liver transplant candidates. Liver Int 2014;34(3):469–76.
48. Khan A, Tansel A, White DL, et al. Efficacy of psychosocial interventions in inducing and maintaining alcohol abstinence in patients with chronic liver disease: a systematic review. Clin Gastroenterol Hepatol 2016;14(2):191–202.e4.
49. Singal AK, Bataller R, Ahn J, et al. ACG clinical guideline: alcoholic liver disease. Am J Gastroenterol 2018;113(2):175–94.
50. Vassallo GA, Tarli C, Rando MM, et al. Liver transplantation in patients with alcoholic liver disease: a retrospective study. Alcohol Alcohol 2017;53(December 2017):1–6.
51. Marot A, Henrion J, Knebel J-F, et al. Alcoholic liver disease confers a worse prognosis than HCV infection and non-alcoholic fatty liver disease among patients with cirrhosis: an observational study. PLoS One 2017;12(10):e0186715.
52. Grąt M, Lewandowski Z, Grąt K, et al. Negative outcomes after liver transplantation in patients with alcoholic liver disease beyond the fifth post-transplant year. Clin Transplant 2014;28(10):1112–20.

53. Cuadrado A, Fábrega E, Casafont F, et al. Alcohol recidivism impairs long-term patient survival after orthotopic liver transplantation for alcoholic liver disease. Liver Transpl 2005;11(4):420–6.

54. Faure S, Herrero A, Jung B, et al. Excessive alcohol consumption after liver transplantation impacts on long-term survival, whatever the primary indication. J Hepatol 2012;57(2):306–12.

55. Jain A, DiMartini A, Kashyap R, Youk A. Long-term follow-up after liver transplantation for alcoholic liver disease under tacrolimus. Transplantation 2000;70(9):1335–42.

56. Conjeevaram HS, Hart J, Lissoos TW, et al. Rapidly progressive liver injury and fatal alcoholic hepatitis occurring after liver transplantation in alcoholic patients. Transplantation 1999;67(12):1562–8. Available at: http://www.ncbi.nlm.nih.gov/pubmed/10401763.

57. Rice JP, Eickhoff J, Agni R, et al. Abusive drinking after liver transplantation is associated with allograft loss and advanced allograft fibrosis. Liver Transpl 2013;19(12):1377–86.

58. Pfitzmann R, Schwenzer J, Rayes N, et al. Long-term survival and predictors of relapse after orthotopic liver transplantation for alcoholic liver disease. Liver Transpl 2007;13(2):197–205.

59. Dumortier J, Dharancy S, Cannesson A, et al. Recurrent alcoholic cirrhosis in severe alcoholic relapse after liver transplantation: a frequent and serious complication. Am J Gastroenterol 2015;110(8):1160–6.

60. DiMartini A, Dew MA, Day N, et al. Trajectories of alcohol consumption following liver transplantation. Am J Transplant 2010;10(10):2305–12.

61. Welzel TM, Graubard BI, El-Serag HB, et al. Risk factors for intrahepatic and extrahepatic cholangiocarcinoma in the United States: a population-based case-control study. Clin Gastroenterol Hepatol 2007;5(10):1221–8.

62. Yen YH, Chang KC, Tsai MC, et al. Elevated body mass index is a risk factor associated with possible liver cirrhosis across different etiologies of chronic liver disease. J Formos Med Assoc 2018;117(4):268–75.

63. Di Stefano C, Vanni E, Mirabella S, et al. Risk factors for arterial hypertension after liver transplantation. J Am Soc Hypertens 2018;12(3):220–9.

64. Wild SH, Walker JJ, Morling JR, et al. Cardiovascular disease, cancer, and mortality among people with type 2 diabetes and alcoholic or nonalcoholic fatty liver disease hospital admission. Diabetes Care 2018;41(2):341–7.

65. Addolorato G, Mirijello A, Leggio L, et al. Liver transplantation in alcoholic patients: impact of an alcohol addiction unit within a liver transplant center. Alcohol Clin Exp Res 2013;37(9):1601–8.

66. Donnadieu-Rigole H, Olive L, Nalpas B, et al. Follow-up of alcohol consumption after liver transplantation: interest of an addiction team? Alcohol Clin Exp Res 2017;41(1):165–70.

67. Heyes CM, Schofield T, Gribble R, et al. Reluctance to accept alcohol treatment by alcoholic liver disease transplant patients. Transplant Direct 2016;2(10):e104.

68. Rodrigue JR, Hanto DW, Curry MP. Substance abuse treatment and its association with relapse to alcohol use after liver transplantation. Liver Transpl 2013;19(12):1387–95.

69. Willenbring ML, Olson DH. A randomized trial of integrated outpatient treatment for medically ill alcoholic men. Arch Intern Med 1999;159(16):1946–52.

70. Crabb DW, Bataller R, Chalasani NP, et al. Standard definitions and common data elements for clinical trials in patients with alcoholic hepatitis: recommendation

from the NIAAA alcoholic hepatitis consortia. Gastroenterology 2016;150(4): 785–90.

71. Hughes E, Hopkins LJ, Parker R. Survival from alcoholic hepatitis has not improved over time. PLoS One 2018;13(2):1–10.

72. Michelena J, Altamirano J, Abraldes JG, et al. Systemic inflammatory response and serum lipopolysaccharide levels predict multiple organ failure and death in alcoholic hepatitis. Hepatology 2015;62(3):762–72.

73. Thursz MR, Richardson P, Allison M, et al. Prednisolone or pentoxifylline for alcoholic hepatitis. N Engl J Med 2015;372(17):1619–28.

74. Vergis N, Atkinson SR, Knapp S, et al. In patients with severe alcoholic hepatitis, prednisolone increases susceptibility to infection and infection-related mortality, and is associated with high circulating levels of bacterial DNA. Gastroenterology 2017;152(5):1068–77.e4.

75. Parker R, Armstrong MJ, Corbett C, et al. Systematic review: pentoxifylline for the treatment of severe alcoholic hepatitis. Aliment Pharmacol Ther 2013;37(9): 845–54.

76. Lee BP, Mehta N, Platt L, et al. Outcomes of early liver transplantation for patients with severe alcoholic hepatitis. Gastroenterology 2018;155(2):422–30.e1.

77. Neuberger J. Public and professional attitudes to transplanting alcoholic patients. Liver Transpl 2007;13(3):S65–8.

78. Stroh G, Rosell T, Dong F, et al. Early liver transplantation for patients with acute alcoholic hepatitis: public views and the effects on organ donation. Am J Transplant 2015;15(6):1598–604.

Chronic Neurologic Effects of Alcohol

Nadia Hammoud, MD[a], Joohi Jimenez-Shahed, MD[b],*

KEYWORDS

- Alcohol • Complications • Wernicke-Korsakoff encephalopathy
- Cerebellar degeneration • Ataxia • Alcoholic neuropathy

KEY POINTS

- The chronic effects of alcohol abuse on the central and peripheral nervous systems can be clinically subtle or profound, but they are usually irreversible.
- Several factors influence the pathophysiology of chronic alcohol abuse, including genetic factors that influence alcohol use and metabolism, and direct and indirect effects of excessive alcohol consumption (eg, nutritional deficits and liver disease).
- The most important intervention that can be provided to prevent further neurologic devastation is early identification and cessation of alcohol abuse.

INTRODUCTION

The effects of chronic alcohol abuse on the nervous system span a spectrum of disorders from acute processes to more chronic, and often irreversible, ones. Such neurologic effects can be seen in both the central and peripheral nervous systems, can be obvious or subtle, and can occur without significant clinical signs to suggest pathologic change. Variables including the quantity of alcohol consumed, age of onset, chronicity of heavy alcohol consumption, and incompletely understood genetic factors; all have been implicated in the neurologic damage that accrues in alcoholics.[1,2]

Acutely, the neurologic effects of alcohol consumption are represented by intoxication, the so-called blackout phenomenon, alcohol-withdrawal–related seizures, and acute myopathy that develop over hours to days.[3] Over time, alcohol abuse is associated with neuropsychological presentations such as withdrawal symptoms (delirium tremens) and hepatic encephalopathy related to decompensated liver cirrhosis. However, independent of liver disease, chronic alcoholics can experience a range of

Disclosures: The authors have nothing to disclose.
[a] Department of Neurology, Baylor College of Medicine, 7200 Cambridge Street, 9th Floor, MS: BCM609, Houston, TX 77030, USA; [b] Department of Neurology, Parkinson's Disease Center and Movement Disorders Clinic, Baylor College of Medicine, 7200 Cambridge Street, 9th Floor, MS: BCM609, Houston, TX 77030, USA
* Corresponding author.
E-mail address: jshahed@bcm.edu

Clin Liver Dis 23 (2019) 141–155
https://doi.org/10.1016/j.cld.2018.09.010
1089-3261/19/© 2018 Elsevier Inc. All rights reserved.

neurologic complications, both cognitive and motor, that can develop in a subacute to chronic time frame. In addition, chronic alcohol use can independently increase the risk for neurovascular disease and depression.[4,5]

The chronic neurologic effects of alcohol affect an estimated 50% of chronic alcohol users.[6] By one study in 1984, in hospitalized chronic alcoholics who were randomly selected at their first admission for detoxification, 68% had cognitive deficits (aside from Wernicke encephalopathy), 74% presented with peripheral neuropathy, and 24% had evidence of autonomic dysregulation, all of which were presumed to be linked to chronic alcohol use. Of these patients, 80% had some degree of liver damage.[7] Although several studies have suggested that women are more susceptible to the neurocognitive effects of alcohol abuse, specific studies that have been designed to compare the global deficits in men and women have been inconclusive.[2]

The effects of alcohol on the nervous system and the long-term pathophysiologic changes that are induced are complicated and mediated both by the direct toxic effects and by the resultant nutritional deficiencies caused by long-standing alcohol use.[1,3,8] On the level of neurotransmission, alcohol affects virtually every major neurotransmitter, as shown in **Table 1**.[1,5] The structural and functional changes that occur in the brains of alcoholics in the absence of clinically identifiable neurologic disease have been referred to as alcohol-related brain damage, which may represent one end of a spectrum of disorders or isolated phenomena that lack clinical correlation.[9] The broader spectrum of alcohol-related neurologic dysfunction (ARND) is similarly complex, with pathophysiologic contributions from both direct and indirect effects of alcohol consumption, as described in **Fig. 1**. It is still unclear whether the genetic features that predispose individuals who develop alcohol dependence or alcoholic liver disease also increase the incidence or risk of ARND.[1,2,8–10]

An emerging mechanism of neurologic injury suggests that alcohol creates significant endoplasmic reticulum stress in the neuroglia leading to the production of stress-response proteins and neurotrophic factor, and initiates the abnormal

Table 1	
Major neurotransmitter systems modulated by chronic alcohol use	
Neurotransmitter	**Effect**
Dopamine	Increased use in the nucleus accumbens, which mediates ethanol's pleasurable and rewarding effects in the mesolimbic system
GABA	Ethanol potentiates GABAergic activity that produces the anxiolytic and ataxic effects, as well as the amnestic and sedative properties of ethanol use
Glutamate	The neurodepressive effects of ethanol arise from blockade of the NMDA receptor, therefore opposing the excitatory effects of glutamate
Noradrenaline	The activating effects of alcohol use arise from the increased release of noradrenaline (norepinephrine) from the locus ceruleus
Opioids	The analgesic, pleasure-inducing, and stress-reducing effects of alcohol are mediated by endogenous opioid release
Serotonin	Ethanol stimulates release of 5HT3 from the raphe nuclei, therefore producing the noxious, nauseating effects of ethanol

Abbreviations: GABA, gamma-aminobutyric acid; 5HT3, 5-hydroxytryptamine; NMDA, N-methyl-D-aspartate.
Data from Mcintosh C, Chick J. Alcohol and the nervous system. J Neurol Neurosurg Psychiatry 2004;75(suppl_3):S16-21.

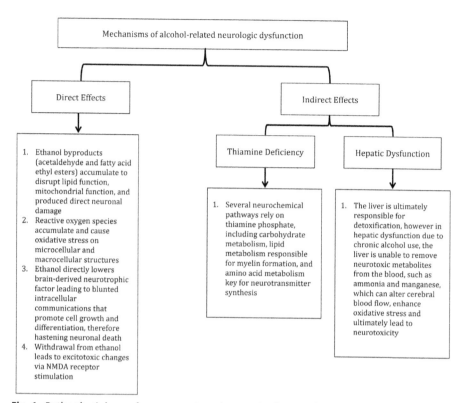

Fig. 1. Pathophysiology of nervous system damage in chronic alcohol use. NMDA, N-methyl-d-aspartate.

phosphorylation of downstream proteins that ultimately lead to neuronal cell death.[2] In addition, chronic alcohol exposure alters the blood-brain barrier in a way that increases the diffusion of alcohol into the central nervous system (CNS) but also increases the passage of inflammatory products and leukocytes. In conjunction with reactive oxygen species, this mediates changes to the endothelium, which then upregulates expression of platelet endothelial cell adhesion molecule 1 (PECAM-1), which then further propagates neuroinflammation.[2]

Neuroinflammation is a result of a complex interplay between systemic inflammation and the nervous system. Heavy alcohol use has been linked to this increased inflammatory response that is predominantly mediated by cytokines: interleukin 1β, interleukin 6, interferon-gamma, and tumor necrosis factor (TNF)-alpha. Changes in the transcription of certain microglial genes occurs during alcohol exposure as these immune cells attempt to re-establish homeostasis in the CNS. Of the proinflammatory markers, TNF-alpha plays a key role in apoptotic cell death and is released from microglial cells. Of note, TNF-alpha production has also been implicated in the pathophysiologic changes responsible for neurodegenerative conditions such as Alzheimer disease, although its specific contribution to neuronal dysfunction and injury is still not fully understood.[2,8,11] Regardless, controlling systemic inflammation (ie, hepatic injury) caused by alcohol may also be an important component to treatment and recovery from ARND by reducing the neuroinflammatory mechanisms contributing to CNS injury and degeneration.

This article discusses 3 common neurologic manifestations of chronic alcohol use, cerebellar ataxia, peripheral neuropathy, and Wernicke-Korsakoff encephalopathy

(WKE), including clinical features, pathogenesis, diagnosis, and potential treatments where available. The objective of this discussion is to inform health care providers and general public on the deleterious effects of alcohol on the nervous system, to create impetus for screening and early intervention, and to show the need to continue to study the effects of alcohol on the nervous system in order to better understand how clinicians can address the morbidity and mortality related to alcoholism.

CEREBELLAR ATAXIA

Cerebellar degeneration is a pathologic term to describe slowly accumulating cerebellar changes caused by alcohol toxicity. Cerebellar degeneration occurs in alcoholics with and without micronutrient deficiencies and is considered the most common CNS complication of chronic alcohol use, affecting an estimated 10% to 25% of alcoholics, with some studies citing a 33% incidence among alcoholics.[3,12–14] **Table 2** provides an overview of the pathogenesis, presentation, diagnosis, and treatment of cerebellar degeneration.[3,8,15–17] Of all the toxic-metabolic insults to the cerebellum, alcohol is the most common cause of cerebellar disease; some studies suggest an onset after 10 years of alcohol abuse.[8,17–20] The effect of alcohol on the cerebellum is graded with the most severe deficits occurring in alcoholics with the longest duration and highest severity of use.[21,22]

Cerebellar ataxia is the clinical correlate to cerebellar degeneration and can have varied features. Truncal ataxia describes an instability and disequilibrium of the trunk that causes body oscillations while seated, and is caused by insults to the cerebellar vermis, although gait and limb ataxias have also been documented. In comparison, limb ataxia (also called appendicular ataxia) in the upper extremity presents with dysdiadochokinesis and dysmetria and is related to cerebellar hemispheric damage or dysfunction. Cerebellar gait ataxia refers to a gait that is wide based with difficulties in tandem step.[8,15,17] The so-called rostral vermis syndrome is most characteristically seen in alcoholics and results in a clinical presentation of a wide-based, ataxic gait and relative absence of appendicular ataxia or other cerebellar signs, such as nystagmus or dysarthria. The differential diagnosis for acquired cerebellar ataxia is extensive, but there are several reversible causes that should be excluded if a clear chronicity of alcohol abuse cannot be established. These causes are listed in **Box 1**.[15,17] Other clinical features that may accompany such forms of cerebellar ataxia include hypotonia, dysarthria, nystagmus, and incoordination.[17,23,24] Some clinicians suggest that the most significant risk factor for developing clinically significant degeneration is the duration of alcohol abuse.[25]

The pathophysiology of alcohol-induced cerebellar degeneration is similar to the broader mechanisms of alcohol-induced CNS damage: direct toxicity and nutrient

Table 2	
The clinical features of cerebellar degeneration secondary to chronic alcohol use	
Alcoholic Cerebellar Degeneration	
Epidemiology	Men>women, incidence peaks in mid-decades of life
Pathogenesis	Direct toxic effect on the cerebellar cortex, specifically Purkinje cells Vitamin deficiency, particularly vitamin B_1
Clinical Presentation	Slowly progressive truncal ataxia with cerebellar gait disturbance (ie, wide-based gait with difficulty in tandem walking)
Diagnosis	Clinical; imaging may show anterior-superior vermian atrophy
Treatment	Alcohol cessation and vitamin B_1 (thiamine) supplementation to slow progression; recovery is incomplete

---

Box 1
The differential diagnosis for acquired ataxias, which can be considered in the evaluation of suspected alcoholic cerebellar degeneration

1. Vascular disease (ie, stroke)

2. Demyelinating disease

3. Toxic
   - Ethanol
   - Chemotherapy
   - Solvents
   - Metals (mercury, lead, bismuth, lithium)
   - Select antiepileptics

4. Infectious
   - Human immunodeficiency virus (HIV)
   - Creutzfeldt-Jakob disease
   - Whipple disease
   - Bickerstaff encephalitis
   - Postinfectious

5. Autoimmune and paraneoplastic disorders

6. Structural/neoplastic disease

---

deficiency–mediated disease.[8,15,17] Thiamine deficiency has a strong correlation with cerebellar gait ataxia, which has been observed in several clinical contexts outside of chronic alcohol abuse; for example, in hyperemesis gravidarum, acquired immunodeficiency syndrome, and malignancy.[20] In addition, the ataxia observed in Wernicke encephalopathy, when caused by thiamine deficiency, usually appears before the cognitive features of the syndrome, suggesting that the cerebellum is particularly sensitive to thiamine deficiency.[18,20,26] Within the cerebellum, the anterior-superior vermis most commonly shows degenerative changes (35%–50%) in chronic alcoholics.[3,8,20] Although the damage occurs to all neuronal layers as well as the white matter, the Purkinje cells are most affected.[3,8,17,20,24,27] Because some studies have documented cerebellar ataxia in well-nourished alcoholics, further mechanisms, aside from thiamine deficiency, must also play a role in the development of cerebellar degeneration.[28]

The diagnosis of cerebellar degeneration is largely clinical. MRI can be used to evaluate for vermian atrophy but is unnecessary (**Fig. 2**).[15] The mainstay of treatment is cessation counseling.[3,15] Ultimately, the identification of the toxic insult is crucial in order to limit ongoing exposure, thereby curtailing further damage. However, once cerebellar degeneration is established, aside from thiamine supplementation, treatment is largely supportive because the damage is irreversible.[3,15]

ALCOHOLIC NEUROPATHY

Neuropathy is the main peripheral nervous system manifestation of chronic alcohol abuse, and its occurrence has been well documented. It is possibly the earliest associated neurologic complication of alcoholism and affects nearly 90% of chronic alcohol users.[3,29] The neuropathy can affect both small and large peripheral nerve fibers, leading to different clinical manifestations.

Small fiber neuropathy affects the small, nociceptive fibers and presents as a painful sensory neuropathy accompanied by paresthesias, with deficits in temperature and pinprick sensation on examination.[30] This pure alcohol-related neuropathy is caused by the direct toxic effects of alcohol, which is postulated to inhibit the retrograde

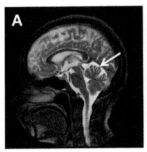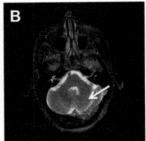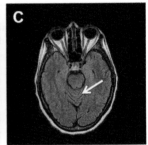

Fig. 2. Cerebellar vermian atrophy in a 52-year old female patient presenting with isolated gait ataxia with mild heel to shin ataxia but no upper extremity involvement, nystagmus, or dysarthria. These findings are typical of alcoholic cerebellar degeneration. (*A*) Sagittal T2-weighted fatsat PROPELLER image showing atrophy of the rostral vermis most prominent in the anterior lobe of the cerebellum (*arrow*). (*B*) Axial T2-weighted fatsat PROPELLER image shows sparing of the cerebellar hemispheres (*arrow*). (*C*) Axial T2 fluid-attenuated inversion recovery (FLAIR) image again reveals superior vermis atrophy (*arrow*).

axonal transport systems of peripheral nerve cells.[3] Thiamine-deficiency–related neuropathy affects larger fiber types, which results in motor deficits and sensory ataxia.[31] On examination, large fiber involvement is manifested by distal limb muscle weakness and loss of proprioception and vibratory sensation. Together, these can contribute to the gait unsteadiness seen in chronic alcoholics by creating a superimposed steppage gait and reduced proprioceptive input back to the movement control loops in the CNS. In chronic alcoholics, both small and large fiber neuropathies can be seen and often present together as a mixed sensorimotor neuropathy.[3]

Chronic alcoholic neuropathy is a length-dependent axonopathy and therefore presents in a so-called stocking-glove pattern. Acutely, patients may report paresthesias and pain, which usually have a slow and progressive onset. As damage accrues, deep tendon reflexes can be lost and proprioceptive losses may develop, which can impair gait. Late symptoms include motor fiber loss and present as weakness and atrophy.[3] Importantly, autonomic dysfunction can ensue because of loss of these fiber types, presenting as orthostasis, incontinence, impotence, and vasomotor dysfunction (**Table 3**).[32]

Diagnosis begins with laboratory evaluation to exclude other causes of distal, sensorimotor neuropathy: hemoglobin A1c, liver function testing, and complete blood count to evaluate for red blood cell macrocytosis are suggested. Cerebrospinal fluid studies may show increased protein levels but should otherwise be normal in cases of alcohol neuropathy and are not recommended in routine evaluation.[3] Electromyography (EMG) and nerve conduction studies (NCS) can be used to distinguish whether the neuropathy is axonal or demyelinating and whether it is motor, sensory, or mixed type. Alcoholic neuropathy shows reduced distal, sensory amplitudes and, to a lesser extent, reduced motor amplitudes on NCS.[3] It is important to remember that small fiber neuropathies may not be measurable on NCS. Skin biopsy can be considered to evaluate specifically for small fiber neuropathy, but nerve biopsy is often not indicated because laboratory and EMG/NCS testing in combination with clinical history is often sufficient to elicit a diagnosis.[3] A limited differential for acquired neuropathies is provided in **Box 2**.[33] The authors recommend that modifiable factors be checked before fully attributing neuropathy in alcoholic patients to an untreatable process.

Treatment of alcoholic peripheral neuropathy is largely targeted at identifying additional nutritional deficiencies and providing supplementation. However, vitamin and

Table 3 The clinical features associated with alcoholic neuropathy	
Pathogenesis	Direct toxicity to the peripheral nerve axon via the retrograde transport system Nutritional deficiency
Clinical Presentation	Slow and progressive Stocking and glove distribution Early symptoms include pain and paresthesias Later symptoms include loss of proprioception, gait disturbance, and loss of reflexes Most advanced findings include weakness and muscle atrophy
Diagnosis	Laboratory testing to exclude other causes of distal axonopathies (HbA1c, LFTs, CBC) Electromyography and nerve conduction stimulation In rare cases skin biopsy to show small fiber loss
Treatment	Alcohol cessation and vitamin supplementation to stop progression In mild to moderate cases, near-complete improvement can be achieved

Abbreviations: CBC, complete blood count; HbA1c, hemoglobin A1c; LFTs, liver function tests.

nutritional supplementation alone is insufficient to stop progression.[3] Alcohol cessation is the cornerstone of treatment, and long-term follow-up is necessary to ensure that patients are compliant. In individuals with mild to moderate neuropathy, a significant but incomplete improvement in symptoms can be achieved. Recovery is unlikely in alcoholics with severe neuropathy at presentation.[3]

WERNICKE-KORSAKOFF ENCEPHALOPATHY

WKE is a 2-part syndrome widely associated with chronic alcohol abuse. Wernicke encephalopathy (WE) alone is 10 times more prevalent in chronic alcohol abusers compared with the general population.[20] Autopsy review suggests that the overall incidence of WE in the western hemisphere is 0.4% to 2.8%.[34] However, in the alcoholic population, that number is increased nearly 6-fold to 12.5%.[35] In an Australian study in 1983, the prevalence of WE was 3:1, affecting men more than women (**Table 4**).[36]

WKE is caused by thiamine deficiency in chronic alcoholics who are malnourished.[3,8] However, there are several other causes of thiamine deficiency that can precipitate WKE.[37] Specifically in Korsakoff syndrome (KS), a genetic component that predisposes individuals to severe amnesia has been proposed. It is possible that these individuals lack enzymes, either because of deficiency or dysfunction, that are important in the metabolism of thiamine or vitamin B_1.[2] The areas of the CNS most commonly affected in WE include the thalamus, mammillary bodies, periaqueductal gray matter and oculomotor regions of the midbrain, and the pons.[38] Some of these same areas are implicated in KS; however, cortical and other subcortical damage plays additional, poorly understood roles in the development of KS.[39]

WE develops acutely, usually over days to weeks, and presents with a triad of altered mental status, gait ataxia, and ophthalmoplegia.[3,8] Only 10% of patients present with all 3 features, with the most common clinical finding being altered mental status and, in extreme cases, coma.[40,41] More specifically, the cognitive changes that can accompany WE include diminished attention, memory impairment, disorientation, and abulia (decreased spontaneous speech).[3] The visual disturbances reported

---

Box 2
A differential diagnosis for alcoholic neuropathy, which is typically a distal, mixed axonopathy

- Endocrine
  - Diabetes mellitus
  - Hypothyroidism

- Infectious
  - HIV
  - Hepatitis
  - Syphilis
  - Leprosy
  - Lyme disease

- Autoimmune
  - Guillain-Barré syndrome

- Neoplastic
  - Lymphoma
  - Carcinoma/paraneoplastic disorders
  - Multiple myeloma

- Systemic
  - Chronic liver disease
  - End-stage renal disease
  - Amyloidosis

- Nutritional
  - Vitamin B_6
  - Vitamin B_{12}
  - Folic acid
  - Copper

- Toxin
  - Lead
  - Mercury
  - Arsenic
  - Gold
  - Organophosphates
  - Tetanus toxin
  - Diphtheria toxin
  - Antibiotics
  - Antiepileptics

- Critical illness neuropathy

Data from Azhary H, Farooq MU, Bhanushali M, et al. Peripheral neuropathy: differential diagnosis and management. Am Fam Physician 2010;81(7):887–92.

---

by patients may be subtle, and examination is key in order to identify oculomotor deficits. Most commonly, horizontal nystagmus can be appreciated, but this is often accompanied by vertical and rotary nystagmus. Cranial nerve 6 palsy can also be appreciated and is usually asymmetric.[3] Gait ataxia is more commonly demonstrated in WE, although truncal ataxia has also been documented. Most importantly, patients with concomitant thiamine neuropathy can have a masked gait ataxia. Irrespective, the treatment is emergent thiamine supplementation for either cause.

Eighty percent of patients with WE progress to develop KS.[37] It is unclear whether WE must precede KS in order for the latter to develop.[3] The association between these two processes was first identified by autopsy, in which the same neuropathologic lesions were described in the same areas of the brain in both diagnosed diseases.[42] KS presents as confabulation, a compensatory response to the inability to recall, as well

Table 4	
The clinical features of Wernicke-Korsakoff encephalopathy	
Epidemiology	Incidence in nonalcoholics is 0.4%–2.8%
	In chronic alcoholics, the incidence is 12.5%
Pathogenesis	Thiamine deficiency
Clinical Presentation	Acute onset
	Gait ataxia
	Ophthalmoplegia with horizontal > vertical or rotary nystagmus
	Cognitive change, including poor attention, memory deficits, disorientation, alogia
	Coma
	Korsakoff confabulation presents with anterograde and retrograde amnesia in the absence of altered sensorium or oculomotor findings
Diagnosis	Primarily clinical
	Blood ketolase levels may be normal in previous thiamine replacement
	FLAIR MRI with diffusion restriction in the thalamus, mammillary bodies, periaqueductal gray and oculomotor region of the midbrain, and pons
Treatment	Thiamine replacement with 1 g of intravenous thiamine every 24 h
	Do not delay initiation of thiamine in order to obtain diagnostic testing
	Memory deficits may take up to 2 y to resolve despite treatment
	Thiamine supplementation addresses confabulation; however, the amnestic features of Korsakoff syndrome are persistent

Abbreviation: FLAIR, fluid-attenuated inversion recovery.

as both a retrograde and anterograde amnesia. Symptomatic treatment usually addresses the confabulatory aspects of KS, but the amnestic findings are more difficult to reverse.[3]

WE requires prompt treatment with thiamine.[3,8] Delay in treatment, especially in order to pursue diagnostic testing, can be fatal, with a 20% mortality.[43] There has been some controversy surrounding thiamine supplementation. Emergently, the recommended dosage for thiamine replacement is 1 g of parenteral thiamine per day with reassessment of levels within 72 hours.[3] Some guidelines previously suggested 100 mg of oral or intramuscular thiamine per day, but it was unclear whether this dose was sufficient to penetrate the CNS.[44,45] It is still widely accepted to supplement with oral thiamine (at least for 1 month) in alcoholic patients who continue to drink, because the side effects of thiamine supplementation are fairly benign.[5,37] Despite treatment, cognitive changes may persist for several years.[43]

KS is a treatable condition, with a quarter of patients showing slight improvement, another quarter showing moderate improvement, and another quarter showing full recovery. Therefore, a quarter of patients with KS develop progressive, irreversible amnesia.[5] There is a significant morbidity associated with KS, with up to 25% of patients requiring institutionalization, despite appropriate thiamine replacement efforts.[46,47] These outcomes are likely related to the fact that patients with KS often have delayed presentation to health care providers, so significant deficits have developed by the time of initial assessment.[5] This finding further bolsters the claim that early screening and cessation efforts are imperative when evaluating patients with alcohol use disorder.

OTHER CONSIDERATIONS
Alcoholic Dementia

Chronic alcohol abuse is strongly linked to neurodegeneration and is thought to contribute to 10% of all cases of dementia.[48] However, some studies suggest that around 25% of all causes of dementia are linked to heavy alcohol use.[49] In a study examining alcohol consumption and cognitive decline, it was determined that excessive alcohol consumption (more than 36 g per day) led to an additional 2 to 6 years of cognitive deficits beyond those associated with age alone.[50] In addition, alcoholic dementia presents earlier than other acquired forms of dementia.[3]

The CNS atrophy that has been linked to alcoholic neurodegeneration is caused by destruction of myelin and loss of dendritic connections as well as neuronal loss.[27] This loss occurs most prominently in the prefrontal regions and corpus callosum, and occurs independently from thiamine deficiency.[8,51] The pattern of decline in alcoholics is progressive in several cognitive domains, which differentiates primary alcoholic dementia from Wernicke-Korsakoff syndrome, which primarily presents as an amnestic phenomenon.[47] Evaluation of alcoholic dementia includes exclusion of reversible causes to assist in providing a definitive diagnosis, if possible.[8] Like the degenerative process discussed previously, cessation can, at best, mildly reverse some of the cognitive deficits, and mainly serves to limit progression. Treatment otherwise remains largely supportive.

Marchiafava-Bignami Syndrome

Of the degenerative disease associated with chronic alcohol use, Marchiafava-Bignami is a syndrome that involves myelin. It presents in an acute and chronic form, and the former can be lethal.[8] The syndrome involves altered mental status, ataxia, mood disorder (depression and mania), and features of psychosis (paranoia).[3,47] Over time, an interhemispheric disconnection syndrome develops that presents with dementia, tactile and unilateral agraphia, limb apraxia, and hemialexia.[52] The primary cause is demyelination of the corpus callosum, specifically the splenium.[8] Demyelination may also extend into the cortical gray matter, optic tracts, subcortical areas, and the cerebellar peduncles.[52] MRI with diffusion-weighted imaging shows widespread involvement of the corpus callosum.[3] It is unclear whether thiamine deficiency also plays a role in this syndrome; it is similar in many aspects to WE, and can occur concomitantly. Therefore, some clinicians suggest that supplementation with thiamine may be beneficial in slowing the progression of Marchiafava-Bignami syndrome.[8]

Alcoholic Myopathy and Combined System Degeneration of the Spinal Cord

Chronic alcoholic myopathy affects an estimated 2% to 5% of adults in the western hemisphere, making this entity one of the most common causes of muscle disease.[53] The prevalence is higher in women.[3] Up to 60% of alcoholics develop muscle disease after an average of 3 years of chronic alcohol use, and the damage is additive.[53,54] Alcoholic myopathy is more common in patients with other sequelae of chronic alcohol-related disease; 50% of cirrhotics have myopathy.[53] Acute forms exist, presenting after episodes of binge drinking with weakness, pain, tenderness, and swelling of affected muscles. Rhabdomyolysis may be present. Symptoms can resolve with alcohol abstinence. Proposed mechanisms of injury in acute and chronic alcoholic myopathy include[53,54]:

1. Direct alcohol toxicity leading to apoptosis
2. Decreased synthetic function as well as dysfunctional protein degradation, specifically myofibrillar and sarcoplasmic proteins

3. Altered cell membrane permeability and function
4. Free radical–mediated injury, specifically in type II fibers
5. Reduction in glycolytic enzymes necessary for lactate production in anaerobic exercise
6. Acetaldehyde-mediated protein adduct formation
7. Loss of muscle progenitor cells

These various mechanisms are proinflammatory and create increased oxidative stress on the cellular level.[53]

Chronic alcoholic myopathy typically presents with painless, proximal weakness accompanied by atrophy that develops over weeks to months.[53] The differential includes glucocorticoid myopathy, hypothyroidism, hypophosphatemia, disuse atrophy, and critical illness myopathy.[3] Histopathologically, atrophy of type IIb fibers can be seen with a non-specific moth-eaten appearance.[3] Neuropathic changes are not seen. Diagnosis is largely made by history, but other causes of myopathy should be excluded. Myoglobinuria is absent and creatinine kinase levels are normal but can also be reduced or marginally increased, especially in the context of an acute myopathy. Cardiomyopathy should be excluded as well. Electrodiagnostic testing can show concomitant neuropathy, as discussed earlier. Like alcoholic neuropathy, mild to moderate clinical cases show the most reversibility with abstinence, with up to 85% of patients achieving improvement in strength within 1 year of cessation. As for other alcohol-related problems, heavier alcohol consumption and more severe symptoms are associated with worse prognosis.[3,53]

Myelopathy is another neurologic complication of chronic alcohol use. First described in patients with decompensated cirrhosis and portal shunting, later studies reported similar clinical findings in patients without evident hepatic dysfunction or malnutrition.[55] Through case reports, it has been speculated that alcoholic injury to the spinal cord is also direct and indirect, via hepatic disease as well as nutritional deficiencies, primarily cobalamin (vitamin B_{12}) and folic acid.[56]

In hepatic myelopathy, which is largely caused by hepatoportal shunting, patients present with a progressive, spastic, hyper-reflexic paresis of the lower extremities. Fluid-attenuated inversion recovery (FLAIR) MRI studies show subcortical and lateral spinal cord tract changes, which correlate with postmortem findings of variable degrees of bilateral, symmetric axonal damage.[57] Case reports of chronic alcoholics without hepatic disease describe the same lateral cord findings but with the additional findings of decreased proprioception and gait abnormalities.[56] This finding supports the potential for a direct toxic effect of alcohol on the spinal cord, which manifests as a combined posterior and lateral column disease. Close monitoring of nutrient levels and appropriate supplementation, and, more importantly, alcohol cessation, are key to halting the progression of both sensory and motor myelopathy.[54,56]

Alcohol abuse poses additional risks that directly affect CNS health, including neurovascular disease and depression. Light to moderate use (ie, less than or equal to 2 drinks per day for men and less than or equal to 1 drink per day for women) has been shown to be neuroprotective against stroke by increasing the levels of healthy high-density lipoprotein. However, in higher concentrations, alcohol has the potential to precipitate cardioembolic events leading to ischemic stroke. It also increases the risk of hemorrhagic stroke via alcohol-induced hypertension and therefore also increases the risk of developing increased intracranial pressures. Active alcoholics are also at higher risk of developing obstructive sleep apnea leading to severe hypoxemia, which itself increases the risk of stroke but also can result in chronic, neurocognitive deficits and mood disorders.[4]

Box 3
Summary of the neurologic complications of chronic alcohol use

1. Cerebellar ataxia
   - Direct toxic effect of ethanol to the cerebellar cortex as well as thiamine deficiency–mediated disease
   - Slowly progressive, presenting with truncal ataxia and cerebellar gait
   - Diagnosis is clinical
   - MRI findings consistent with vermian atrophy
   - Treat with thiamine supplementation; however, incomplete recovery

2. Alcoholic neuropathy
   - Progressive mixed axonopathy that develops in a glove-stocking distribution
   - Caused by direct axonal toxicity as well as nutritional deficiency
   - Early symptoms include pain and paresthesias or numbness, which, if left unaddressed, can progress to proprioceptive loss and gait disturbance; in advanced disease, weakness and muscle atrophy can be seen
   - Diagnosis involves exclusion of other acquired neuropathies and cessation is imperative for recovery
   - Recovery is incomplete at best, with the best prognosis reserved for mild disease

3. Wernicke-Korsakoff encephalopathy
   - Strong correlation to chronic alcohol abuse
   - Secondary to thiamine deficiency
   - Acute onset of altered mental status, ophthalmoplegia and gait ataxia; Korsakoff confabulation with anterograde and retrograde amnesia
   - Diagnosis is clinical; however, MRI signal abnormalities can be seen in the mamillary bodies and periaqueductal gray matter
   - Treatment with prompt thiamine administration (1g/24 h parenterally with reevaluation at 72 hours) can reverse Wernicke encephalitis; amnesia is permanent in Korsakoff syndrome

4. Other considerations
   - Alcoholic dementia presents with deficits in multiple cognitive domains and is a common cause of dementia
   - Marchiafava-Bignami syndrome is a demyelinating disease of the corpus callosum and presents in an acute, potentially fatal form as well as a chronic form associated with interhemispheric disconnection
   - Alcoholic myelopathy is secondary to direct and indirect effects of alcohol (vitamin B_{12} and folate deficiency) and can present with dorsal column signs (loss of proprioception, gait instability, paresthesias) and lateral column signs (spastic paresis and hyper-reflexia); it is distinct from hepatic myelopathy, which is caused by hepatoportal shunting
   - Chronic alcohol use directly and indirectly impacts cerebrovascular health and increases risk of stroke

Risk for developing these conditions should be recognized early and patients should be counseled about alcohol cessation, because the process of alcohol-related neurologic dysfunction likely begins before clinical manifestations.

SUMMARY

Chronic alcohol use can induce silent changes in the structure and function of the central and peripheral nervous systems, eventually resulting in irreversible and debilitating repercussions. **Box 3** summarizes the key points discussed throughout this article. Early identification and intervention against alcohol abuse is the most significant step that health care providers can take in order to avoid neurologic complications of chronic alcohol abuse. If disease has already been identified, nutritional supplementation and cessation measures are critical in preventing further damage but may also yield some improvements in symptoms. In individuals with cognitive changes, it is also prudent to identify any cerebellar or motor deficits, because alcohol does not affect 1 area of the nervous system in an isolated manner. In patients with chronic neurologic dysfunction as a result of alcohol use, the prognosis is poor, and supportive measures are the mainstay of management. The proposed mechanisms of neurologic injury in chronic alcohol abuse include direct and indirect toxic effects of alcohol, including hepatic dysfunction; nutritional deficiencies; and, importantly, systemic inflammation that initiates a neuroinflammatory cascade. It remains unclear what benefit may be gained by current standards of management of hepatic disease in limiting, or possibly reversing, the neurologic effects of chronic alcohol use. Efforts to record and measure the effects of alcohol on the brain have been limited by a lack of direct tissue studies. It is imperative to continue to explore these mechanisms in order to discover adjunctive approaches to manage or limit these irreversible devastations to the nervous system.

REFERENCES

1. Mukherjee S. Alcoholism and its effects on the central nervous system. Curr Neurovasc Res 2013;10(3):256–62.
2. Obad A, Peeran A, Little JI, et al. Alcohol-mediated organ damages: heart and brain. Front Pharmacol 2018;9:81.
3. Noble JM, Weimer LH. Neurologic complications of alcoholism. Continuum (Minneap Minn) 2014;20:624–41.
4. Daroff RB, Jankovic J, Mazziotta JC, et al. Ischemic cerebrovascular disease. In: Bradley's neurology in clinical practice. vol. 2. 7th edition. London: Elsevier; 2016. p. 920–67.
5. Mcintosh C, Chick J. Alcohol and the nervous system. J Neurol Neurosurg Psychiatry 2004;75(suppl_3):iii16–21.
6. Fama R, Berre A-PL, Hardcastle C, et al. Neurological, nutritional and alcohol consumption factors underlie cognitive and motor deficits in chronic alcoholism. Addict Biol 2017. https://doi.org/10.1111/adb.12584.
7. Franceschi M, Truci G, Comi G, et al. Cognitive deficits and their relationship to other neurological complications in chronic alcoholic patients. J Neurol Neurosurg Psychiatry 1984;47(10):1134–7.
8. Costin B, Miles M. Molecular and neurologic responses to chronic alcohol use. Handb Clin Neurol 2014;125:157–71.
9. Zahr NM, Kaufman KL, Harper CG. Clinical and pathological features of alcohol-related brain damage. Nat Rev Neurol 2011;7(5):284–94.
10. Harper C, Matsumoto I. Ethanol and brain damage. Curr Opin Pharmacol 2005; 5(1):73–8.
11. McCarthy GM, Farris SP, Blednov YA, et al. Microglial-specific transcriptome changes following chronic alcohol consumption. Neuropharmacology 2018; 128:416–24.
12. Lindboe CF, Løberg EM. The frequency of brain lesions in alcoholics. J Neurol Sci 1988;88(1–3):107–13.
13. Yokota O, Tsuchiya K, Terada S, et al. Frequency and clinicopathological characteristics of alcoholic cerebellar degeneration in Japan: a cross-sectional study of 1,509 postmortems. Acta Neuropathol 2006;112(1):43–51.
14. Welch KA. Neurological complications of alcohol and misuse of drugs. Pract Neurol 2011;11(4):206–19.
15. Daroff RB, Jankovic J, Mazziotta JC, et al. Deficiency diseases of the nervous system. In: Yuen T, editor. Bradley's neurology in clinical practice. vol. 2. 7th edition. London: Elsevier; 2016. p. 1226–36.

16. Harper C. The neuropathology of alcohol-related brain damage. Alcohol Alcohol 2009;44(2):136–40.
17. Alekseeva N, McGee J, Kelley RE, et al. Toxic-metabolic, nutritional, and medicinal-induced disorders of cerebellum. Neurol Clin 2014;32(4):901–11.
18. Baker K, Harding A, Halliday G, et al. Neuronal loss in functional zones of the cerebellum of chronic alcoholics with and without Wernickes encephalopathy. Neuroscience 1999;91(2):429–38.
19. Andersen BB. Reduction of Purkinje cell volume in cerebellum of alcoholics. Brain Res 2004;1007(1–2):10–8.
20. Mulholland PJ. Susceptibility of the cerebellum to thiamine deficiency. Cerebellum 2006;5(1):55–63.
21. Sullivan EV, Deshmukh A, Desmond JE, et al. Cerebellar volume decline in normal aging, alcoholism, and Korsakoffs syndrome: relation to ataxia. Neuropsychology 2000;14(3):341–52.
22. Sullivan EV, Pfefferbaum A. Neuroimaging of the Wernicke-Korsakoff syndrome. Alcohol Alcohol 2009;44(2):155–65.
23. Diener HC, Dichgans J, Bacher M, et al. Improvement of ataxia in alcoholic cerebellar atrophy through alcohol abstinence. J Neurol 1984;231(5):258–62.
24. Johnson-Greene D, Adams KM, Gilman S, et al. Impaired upper limb coordination in alcoholic cerebellar degeneration. Arch Neurol 1997;54(4):436–9.
25. Fitzpatrick LE, Jackson M, Crowe SF. Characterization of cerebellar ataxia in chronic alcoholics using the International Cooperative Ataxia Rating Scale (ICARS). Alcohol Clin Exp Res 2012;36(11):1942–51.
26. Butterworth RF. Pathophysiology of alcoholic brain damage: synergistic effects of ethanol, thiamine deficiency and alcoholic liver disease. Metab Brain Dis 1995;10(1):1–8.
27. Harper C, Dixon G, Sheedy D, et al. Neuropathological alterations in alcoholic brains. Studies arising from the New South Wales Tissue Resource Centre. Prog Neuropsychopharmacol Biol Psychiatry 2003;27(6):951–61.
28. Nicolas J, Fernandez-Sola J, Robert J, et al. High ethanol intake and malnutrition in alcoholic cerebellar shrinkage. QJM 2000;93(7):449–56.
29. Vittadini G, Cuonocore M, Colli G, et al. Alcoholic polyneuropathy: a clinical and epidemiological study. Alcohol Alcohol 2001;36(5):393–400.
30. Koike H, Iijima M, Sugiura M, et al. Alcoholic neuropathy is clinicopathologically distinct from thiamine-deficiency neuropathy. Ann Neurol 2003;54(1):19–29.
31. Mellion M, Gilchrist JM, Monte SDL. Alcohol-related peripheral neuropathy: nutritional, toxic, or both? Muscle Nerve 2011;43(3):309–16.
32. Monforte R, Estruch R, Valle-Sole J, et al. Autonomic and peripheral neuropathies in patients with chronic alcoholism. Arch Neurol 1995;52(1):45–51.
33. Azhary H, Farooq MU, Bhanushali M, et al. Peripheral neuropathy: differential diagnosis and management. Am Fam Physician 2010;81(7):887–92. Available at: https://www.aafp.org/afp/2010/0401/p887.html.
34. Harper C, Fornes P, Duyckaerts C, et al. An international perspective on the prevalence of the Wernicke-Korsakoff syndrome. Metab Brain Dis 1995;10(1):17–24.
35. Torvik A. Brain lesions in alcoholics: neuropathological observations. Acta Med Scand 2009;221(S717):47–54.
36. Harper C. The incidence of Wernickes encephalopathy in Australia–a neuropathological study of 131 cases. J Neurol Neurosurg Psychiatry 1983;46(7):593–8.
37. Donnino MW, Vega J, Miller J, et al. Myths and misconceptions of Wernicke's encephalopathy: what every emergency physician should know. Ann Emerg Med 2007;50(6):715–21.

38. Zuccoli G, Santa Cruz D, Bertolini M, et al. MR imaging findings in 56 patients with Wernicke encephalopathy: nonalcoholics may differ from alcoholics. AJNR Am J Neuroradiol 2009;30(1):171–6.
39. Kril JJ, Harper CG. Neuroanatomy and neuropathology associated with Korsakoff's syndrome. Neuropsychol Rev 2012;22(2):72–80.
40. Torvik A, Lindboe CF, Rogde S. Brain lesions in alcoholics. J Neurol Sci 1982; 56(2–3):233–48.
41. Harper CG, Giles M, Finlay-Jones R. Clinical signs in the Wernicke-Korsakoff complex: a retrospective analysis of 131 cases diagnosed at necropsy. J Neurol Neurosurg Psychiatry 1986;49(4):341–5.
42. Malamud N. Relationship between the Wernicke and the Korsakoff syndrome. AMA Arch Neurol Psychiatry 1956;76(6):585.
43. Thomson AD, Marshall EJ. The natural history and pathophysiology of Wernicke's encephalopathy and Korsakoff's psychosis. Alcohol Alcohol 2006;41(2):151–8.
44. Chataway J, Hardman E. Thiamine in Wernickes syndrome–how much and how long? Postgrad Med J 1995;71(834):249.
45. Cook CCH, Hallwood PM, Thomson AD. B vitamin deficiency and neuropsychiatric syndromes in alcohol misuse. Alcohol Alcohol 1998;33(4):317–36.
46. Todd KG, Hazell AS, Butterworth RF. Alcohol-thiamine interactions: an update on the pathogenesis of Wernicke encephalopathy. Addict Biol 1999;4(3):261–72.
47. Brust J. Ethanol and cognition: indirect effects, neurotoxicity and neuroprotection: a review. Int J Environ Res Public Health 2010;7(4):1540–57.
48. Gupta S, Warner J. Alcohol-related dementia: a 21st-century silent epidemic? Br J Psychiatry 2008;193(05):351–3.
49. Smith DM, Atkinson RM. Alcoholism and dementia. Int J Addict 1995;30(13–14): 1843–69.
50. Sabia S, Elbaz A, Britton A, et al. Alcohol consumption and cognitive decline in early old age. Neurology 2014;82(4):332–9.
51. Pfefferbaum A, Sullivan EV. Disruption of brain white matter microstructure by excessive intracellular and extra-cellular fluid in alcoholism: evidence from diffusion tensor imaging. Neuropsychopharmacology 2005;30:423–32.
52. Kim M-J, Kim J-K, Yoo B-G, et al. Acute Marchiafava-Bignami disease with widespread callosal and cortical lesions. J Korean Med Sci 2007;22(5):908.
53. Simon L, Jolley SE, Molina PE. Alcoholic myopathy: pathophysiologic mechanisms and clinical implications. Alcohol Res 2017;38(2):207–17.
54. Preedy VR, Adachi J, Ueno Y, et al. Alcoholic skeletal muscle myopathy: definitions, features, contribution of neuropathy, impact and diagnosis. Eur J Neurol 2001;8(6):677–87.
55. Sage JI, Van Uitert RL, Lepore FE. Alcoholic myelopathy without substantial liver disease. Arch Neurol 1984;41(9):999.
56. Koike H, Nakamura T, Ikeda S, et al. Alcoholic myelopathy and nutritional deficiency. Intern Med 2017;56(1):105–8.
57. De la Monte SM, Kril JJ. Human alcohol-related neuropathology. Acta Neuropathol 2013;127(1):71–90.

Will Studies in Nonalcoholic Steatohepatitis Help Manage Alcoholic Steatohepatitis?

Vinay Sundaram, MD, MSc[a], Timothy R. Morgan, MD[b],*

KEYWORDS

- Alcoholic cirrhosis • Fatty liver disease • Alcoholic liver disease • Anti-fibrotic
- Anti-inflammatory

KEY POINTS

- Among patients with severe alcoholic hepatitis, the only medication that has been consistently demonstrated to increase short-term survival is corticosteroids.
- Among nonresponders to corticosteroid treatment, mortality ranges from 70% to 80%, and second-line treatment options do not exist.
- At this moment, there are no approved treatments for nonalcoholic steatohepatitis (NASH), although numerous molecules are under investigation in phase 2 and phase 3 clinical studies, targeting pathways including inflammation, oxidative stress, fibrosis, and cell death. It is feasible that potential treatments for NASH may also aid in treating alcoholic hepatitis, given the physiologic similarities between the two diseases.

INTRODUCTION

Alcohol use disorder remains one of the commonest causes of both acute and chronic liver disease in the United States.[1] Excessive alcohol consumption is the third leading preventable cause of death in the United States, with alcoholic liver disease (ALD) causing nearly 46% of cirrhosis-related deaths.[2] Nearly everyone with alcohol use disorder has steatosis but only a subset of these patients develops alcoholic hepatitis (AH), characterized by hepatocellular damage, including hepatocyte ballooning, Mallory-Denk bodies, and neutrophilic infiltrate; these histologic changes characteristic of AH usually occur over a period of years to decades.[3,4] Until it reaches

Disclosure: The authors have nothing to disclose.
Supported in part by a grant from the National Institute on Alcohol Abuse and Alcoholism (U01 AA 21886) to Dr T.R. Morgan.
[a] Department of Medicine, Comprehensive Transplant Center, Cedars-Sinai Medical Center, 8900 Beverly Boulevard, Suite 250, Los Angeles, CA 90048, USA; [b] Gastroenterology Section, VA Long Beach Healthcare System, 5901 East Seventh Street – 11G, Long Beach, CA 90822, USA
* Corresponding author.
E-mail address: Timothy.morgan@va.gov

advanced stages, ALD is often asymptomatic. ASH is a histologic definition that can occur without clinical manifestations or can present with a syndrome of acute jaundice, known as AH.[2]

Despite the potentially high mortality associated with AH,[2] treatment has not evolved beyond the use of corticosteroids, such as prednisolone.[5] Unfortunately, not all patients respond to prednisolone[6]; thus, novel targeted therapies are urgently needed. Liver transplantation in highly selected AH patients improves survival,[7,8] but several concerns exist that limit the use of this intervention, in particular, lack of standardized policies across transplant centers and validated tools to assess alcohol relapse risk after liver transplantation. Therefore, development of additional pharmacologic therapies is imperative to improve survival among those with severe AH.

This article reviews several mechanisms in the development of steatohepatitis, highlighting mechanistic similarities and differences between ASH and NASH. Additionally, multiple therapies for NASH currently under investigation are reviewed, which may aid in the treatment of ASH, based on common physiologic pathways between ASH and NASH (**Fig. 1**).

IMMUNE SYSTEM AND GUT MICROBIOME

The immune system can be classified into the innate immune system, involving neutrophils, macrophages, and natural killer (NK) cells, and the adaptive immune system, mediated by T cells and B cells.[9] The innate immune system plays a significant role in the early development of both steatosis and steatohepatitis. In particular, both macrophages and Kupffer cells produce proinflammatory and anti-inflammatory cytokines

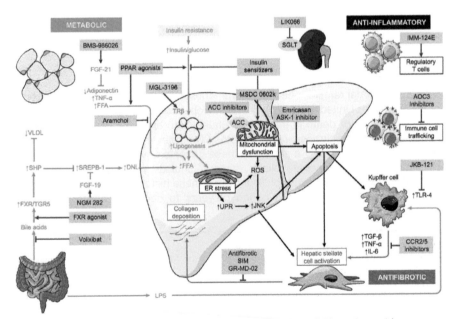

Fig. 1. Potential therapeutic targets for treatment of NASH. AOC3, amine oxidase, copper containing 3; FGF, fibroblast growth factor; IL, interleukin; PPAR, peroxisome proliferator-activated receptor; SGLT, sodium glucose transport protein; SHP, small heterodimer partner; SREBP, sterol regulatory element-binding protein; TGF, transforming growth factor; TLR, toll-like receptor; VLDL, very low density lipoproten.

and activate stellate cells via interleukin (IL)-6 and transforming growth factor β.[9] Consequently, animal models of both ASH and metabolic steatohepatitis have demonstrated that Kupffer cell depletion can reduce hepatic damage and inflammation.[10,11] The innate immune system has an additional role regarding neutrophilic infiltration of the liver, a hallmark of both ASH and NASH.[10–15]

The adaptive immune system plays a prominent role in the later and more advanced stages of ASH and NASH. AH patients develop T-cell infiltration of the liver, in particular helper T cells, and increased circulation of antibodies against lipid peroxidation adducts.[10,16,17] Adaptive immune responses also contribute to hepatic inflammation in NASH,[18] as demonstrated in mouse models showing a decrease of CD4[+] regulatory T cells and secretion of IL-17 by helper T cells, leading to neutrophil chemotaxis.[19,20] T cells also activate stellate cells, which promote collagen deposition in the liver and act as antigen-presenting cells to further stimulate T-cell activity, including NK T cells and CD4[+] and CD8[+] T cells.[21] Inflammatory mediators from both the innate and adaptive immune system are, therefore, potential targets for therapeutic intervention.

Beyond the innate and adaptive immune systems, gut microbiome dysbiosis also may be a therapeutic target for the treatment of alcohol-induced or metabolic steatohepatitis. Prolonged alcohol intake disrupts tight junction proteins and increases gut permeability, thereby allowing for increased endotoxin release into the portal circulation, which is further augmented by overgrowth of gram-negative bacteria.[22] Endotoxin then stimulates the production of tumor necrosis factor (TNF) and other proinflammatory cytokines through activation of Toll-like receptor (TLR) 4 signaling. Other bacteria-derived toxins, such as peptidoglycan and flagellin, may also have an impact on TLR signaling and proinflammatory cytokine production.[23] Endotoxin seems to have role in both steatosis development and hepatic fibrosis.[24]

Data from animal studies also support the notion that gut bacterial dysbiosis may be an important factor in causing NASH through mechanisms of deregulating energy homeostasis,[25] modulation of choline[25] and bile acid metabolism,[26] and generation of bacteria-derived toxins, such as lipopolysaccharide (LPS).[27] Similar to ASH, gut flora may additionally facilitate progression from the simple steatosis to NASH via increased bacterial endotoxin production, thereby leading to increased hepatic TNF-α expression through TLR4 stimulaton.[28] The gut microbiota may also contribute to hepatic fibrosis via stimulation of TLR9-dependent profibrotic pathways in hepatic Kupffer cells.[29]

THERAPIES UNDER INVESTIGATION

IMM-124e is an IgG-rich extract to bovine colostrum from cows immunized against LPS, which can reduce hepatic exposure to gut-derived bacterial toxins. In an open-label, phase 1/2 clinical trial in 10 patients with biopsy-proved NASH, IMM-124e improved liver enzymes as well as glycemic control via increase in serum levels of glucagon-like peptide-1, adiponectin, and regulatory T cells.[30] A phase 2 study of IMM-124e for 24 weeks is ongoing for NASH patients (NCT02316717).

Solithromycin is a next-generation macrolide antibiotic. In a phase 2 open-label study, 6 patients with biopsy-proved NASH (100%) had reductions in nonalcoholic fatty liver disease (NAFLD) activity score (NAS) and alanine aminotransferase level after 90 days of treatment with solithromycin (NCT02510599).[31]

JKB-121 is a long-acting molecule that functions as an antagonist of TLR4. In vitro, JKB-121 neutralized or reduced the LPS-induced release of inflammatory cytokines, deactivated hepatic stellate cells, and inhibited hepatic stellate cell proliferation and collagen expression.[32] A phase 2 trial of JKB-121 for the treatment of NASH is ongoing (NCT02442687).

OXIDATIVE AND ENDOPLASMIC RETICULUM STRESS

Oxidative stress is due to the imbalance between prooxidants and antioxidants. Reactive oxygen species and reactive nitrogen species are beneficial products of normal metabolism.[33] Overproduction of reactive oxygen species and reactive nitrogen species, however, in the setting of inadequate antioxidants can lead to liver injury through both direct cell injury and cell signaling, such as via nuclear factor κB, subsequently leading to production of proinflammatory cytokines.[3]

Endoplasmic reticulum (ER) stress is activated by conditions of protein overload or increased unfolded proteins, which over a prolonged period of time can ultimately result in cell death. Increasing evidence has demonstrates that ER stress is a common feature of many liver diseases, including ASH[34,35] and NASH.[36] Mechanisms that cause ER stress in NAFLD include excess fatty acids, oxidative stress, impaired hepatic autophagy and down-regulation of adiponectin.[37–39] Several alcohol-driven factors are also known to cause ER stress, including acetaldehyde and toxic lipid-derived aldehydes and metabolites, oxidative stress, dysregulated methionine metabolism, and disruption of calcium homeostasis.[40,41]

THERAPIES UNDER INVESTIGATION

Acetyl–coenzyme A (CoA) carboxylase (ACC) is a key enzyme that regulates the conversion of malonyl-CoA to acetyl-CoA.[42] Therefore, inhibition of ACC increases levels of malonyl-CoA, which subsequently increases fatty acid metabolism. GS-0976 is an ACC inhibitor that has been evaluated in an open-label proof-of-concept study in NASH patients.[31,43] Among 10 patients treated with GS-0976 for 12 weeks, there was significant improvement in liver fat content and noninvasive markers of fibrosis. Additionally, patients saw a 43% median relative decrease in liver fat content, from 15.7% to 9.0% ($P = .006$), as measured by MRI–proton density fat fraction and reduction in median liver stiffness from 3.4 kPa to 3.1 kPa at week 12 ($P = .049$), as determined by magnetic resonance elastography. A separate phase 2 study evaluating GS-0976 in 126 patients with NASH has been completed.[31]

Obeticholic acid is a farnesoid X receptor (FXR) agonist, currently approved for treatment of primary biliary cholangitis. FXR agonism engages in a negative feedback loop for bile acid homeostasis that decreases lipogenesis and increases fatty acid oxidation.[44] This can potentially counteract the development of steatosis in NASH and ASH. Additionally, FXR activation may down-regulate stellate cell activation, therefore also functioning as an antifibrotic agent.[45] Currently, FXR agonist studies are still under way for both NASH and ASH.

FIBROSIS AND CELL DEATH

Fibrosis results from an imbalance between production and resorption of extracellular matrix. Stellate cells are the main contributors to fibrosis, which on activation produce profibrogenic factors, such as collagen and smooth muscle actin.[46] Hepatic injury often involves dysregulation of the fibrin cascade, resulting in the formation of fibrin clots that can lead to hepatocellular death. Inhibition of fibrinolysis by plasminogen activator inhibitor-1 (PAI-1) can cause fibrin–extracellular matrix to accumulate in the liver; this imbalance of elevated PAI-1 levels and subsequent hypofibrinolysis is commonly seen in patients with both NASH and ASH.[47] It has been shown that rising plasma PAI-1 levels correlate with worsening hepatic steatosis.[48]

The mechanisms of cell death in all etiologies of liver disease are primarily related to apoptosis and necrosis.[49] Apoptosis and necrosis frequently coexist in liver disease, with necrosis tending to be more dominant in ASH and apoptosis in NASH.

THERAPIES UNDER INVESTIGATION

Cenicriviroc (CVC), a C–C motif chemokine receptor-2/5 (CCR2/5) antagonist, has been developed to primarily target inflammation, but also has antifibrotic effects.[50] CCR5 antagonism, in particular, impairs the migration, activation, and proliferation of hepatic stellate cells.[51] Data from the phase 2b CENTAUR study demonstrated improvement of fibrosis without worsening NASH after 1 year of CVC treatment in 20% of patients receiving CVC compared with 10% of those taking placebo.[52] Phase 3 evaluation for the treatment of NASH with stage 2/3 fibrosis is ongoing and recruiting (AURORA study; NCT03028740).

Selonsertib (GS-4997) is an inhibitor of apoptosis signal-regulating kinase 1 (ASK1), which is activated by extracellular TNF-α or intracellular oxidative/ER stress and subsequently initiates the p38/c-Jun N-terminal kinase (JNK) pathway, resulting in apoptosis and fibrosis.[53] Inhibition of ASK1, therefore, has been proposed as a target for the treatment of NASH and ASH. An open-label phase 2 trial in NASH patients with moderate to severe fibrosis, evaluating selonsertib alone or in combination with the monoclonal antibody against lysyl oxidase-like 2 (LOXL-2) simtuzumab (SIM), has been recently completed. The data demonstrate regression in fibrosis in patients treated with selonsertib for 24 weeks. Patients receiving selonsertib further demonstrated improvements in progression to cirrhosis, liver stiffness, and liver fat content.[54] Phase 3 trials evaluating selonsertib among NASH patients with stage 3 (STELLAR3; NCT03053050) or cirrhosis (STELLAR4; NCT03053063) are ongoing. SIM did not provide additional benefit over selonsertib and, therefore, is no longer under investigation for NASH treatment.[55]

Galectin-3 protein expression, which is essential to the development of hepatic fibrosis, is increased in NASH, with the highest expression in macrophages surrounding lipid-laden hepatocytes. In mouse models, GR-MD-02, a galectin-3 inhibitor, resulted in improved liver histology with a significant reduction in NASH activity and collagen deposition.[56] In phase 2a trials in NASH patients with stage 3 fibrosis, however, there was no significant improvement in fibrosis stage.[57] A phase 2b clinical trial to evaluate the safety and efficacy of GR-MD-02 for the treatment of liver fibrosis and portal hypertension in 162 patients with NASH cirrhosis (NASH-CX trial) is ongoing (NCT02462967).

ND-LO2-s0201 is a vitamin A–coupled lipid nanoparticle containing small interfering RNA against heat shock protein 47, a collagen-specific molecular chaperone needed for the maturation and secretion of collagen. A phase 1 open study is completed to evaluate in subjects with severe hepatic fibrosis (stage 3/4) (NCT02227459).[31]

MN-001 (tipelukast) is a novel, orally bioavailable small-molecule compound that produces antifibrotic and anti-inflammatory activity, including leukotriene receptor antagonism, inhibition of phosphodiesterases 3 and 4, and inhibition of 5-lipoxygenase. An open-label study to evaluate the efficacy, safety, tolerability, and pharmacokinetic tipelukast on high-density lipoprotein function and serum triglyceride levels in NASH/NAFLD with hypertriglyceridemia is ongoing (NCT02681055).[31]

Emricasan, an irreversible caspase inhibitor, improves NAS and fibrosis in murine models of NASH.[58] A phase 2b study in patients with NASH is evaluating the efficacy of 72 weeks of emricasan, 10 mg or 100 mg (ENCORE-NF, NCT02686762). Another phase 2b study in patients with NASH with cirrhosis and severe portal hypertension is assessing the efficacy of 3 doses of emricasan on portal hypertension (ENCORE-PH, NCT02960204), to determine if treatment can reduce hepatic venous pressure gradient.

The adhesion molecule, vascular adhesion protein 1 (VAP-1), is a membrane-bound amine oxidase that promotes leukocyte recruitment to the liver, and the soluble form (sVAP-1) accounts for most circulating monoamine oxidase activity, has insulin-like effects, and can initiate oxidative stress.[59] VAP-1 is directly involved in stellate cell activation and is a strong profibrogenic stimulus. Thus, targeting VAP-1 may result in decreased leukocyte recruitment and reduction of inflammation and fibrosis. BI 1467335 is a VAP-1 inhibitor that works by blocking leukocyte adhesion and tissue infiltration in inflammatory process. Phase 2a of BI 1467335 is a multicenter trial in 150 patients with clinical evidence of NASH (NCT03166735).[31]

SUMMARY

Among patients with severe AH, the only medications that has been consistently demonstrated to increase short-term survival are corticosteroids. Among nonresponders to corticosteroid treatment, however, mortality ranges from 70% to 80%, and second-line treatment options do not exist. At this moment, there are no approved treatments for NASH, although numerous molecules are under investigation in phase 2 and phase 3 clinical studies, targeting pathways, including inflammation, oxidative stress, fibrosis, and cell death. Given the common pathways in the pathogenesis of NASH and ASH, the authors hope that these new agents can be applied to the treatment of severe AH in combination or as a second-line agent to corticosteroids.

REFERENCES

1. Sofair AN, Barry V, Manos MM, et al. The epidemiology and clinical characteristics of patients with newly diagnosed alcohol-related liver disease: results from population-based surveillance. J Clin Gastroenterol 2010;44:301–7.

2. Singal AK, Bataller R, Ahn J, et al. ACG clinical guideline: alcoholic liver disease. Am J Gastroenterol 2018;113:175–94.

3. Joshi-Barve S, Kirpich I, Cave MC, et al. Alcoholic, nonalcoholic, and toxicant-associated steatohepatitis: mechanistic similarities and differences. Cell Mol Gastroenterol Hepatol 2015;1:356–67.

4. Rubin E, Lieber CS. Alcohol-induced hepatic injury in nonalcoholic volunteers. N Engl J Med 1968;278:869–76.

5. Thursz MR, Forrest EH, Ryder S, STOPAH Investigators, et al. Prednisolone or pentoxifylline for alcoholic hepatitis. N Engl J Med 2015;373:282–3.

6. Louvet A, Naveau S, Abdelnour M, et al. The Lille model: a new tool for therapeutic strategy in patients with severe alcoholic hepatitis treated with steroids. Hepatology 2007;45:1348–54.

7. Lee BP, Mehta N, Platt L, et al. Outcomes of early liver transplantation for patients with severe alcoholic hepatitis. Gastroenterology 2018;155(2):422–30.e1.

8. Mathurin P, Moreno C, Samuel D, et al. Early liver transplantation for severe alcoholic hepatitis. N Engl J Med 2011;365:1790–800.

9. Leroux A, Ferrere G, Godie V, et al. Toxic lipids stored by Kupffer cells correlates with their pro-inflammatory phenotype at an early stage of steatohepatitis. J Hepatol 2012;57:141–9.

10. Miura K, Yang L, van Rooijen N, et al. Hepatic recruitment of macrophages promotes nonalcoholic steatohepatitis through CCR2. Am J Physiol Gastrointest Liver Physiol 2012;302:G1310–21.

11. Owumi SE, Corthals SM, Uwaifo AO, et al. Depletion of Kupffer cells modulates ethanol-induced hepatocyte DNA synthesis in C57Bl/6 mice. Environ Toxicol 2014;29:867–75.

12. Alkhouri N, Morris-Stiff G, Campbell C, et al. Neutrophil to lymphocyte ratio: a new marker for predicting steatohepatitis and fibrosis in patients with nonalcoholic fatty liver disease. Liver Int 2012;32:297–302.

13. Dominguez M, Miquel R, Colmenero J, et al. Hepatic expression of CXC chemokines predicts portal hypertension and survival in patients with alcoholic hepatitis. Gastroenterology 2009;136:1639–50.

14. Ibusuki R, Uto H, Arima S, et al. Transgenic expression of human neutrophil peptide-1 enhances hepatic fibrosis in mice fed a choline-deficient, L-amino acid-defined diet. Liver Int 2013;33:1549–56.

15. Joka D, Wahl K, Moeller S, et al. Prospective biopsy-controlled evaluation of cell death biomarkers for prediction of liver fibrosis and nonalcoholic steatohepatitis. Hepatology 2012;55:455–64.

16. Tajiri K, Shimizu Y, Tsuneyama K, et al. Role of liver-infiltrating CD3+CD56+ natural killer T cells in the pathogenesis of nonalcoholic fatty liver disease. Eur J Gastroenterol Hepatol 2009;21:673–80.

17. Thiele GM, Duryee MJ, Willis MS, et al. Autoimmune hepatitis induced by syngeneic liver cytosolic proteins biotransformed by alcohol metabolites. Alcohol Clin Exp Res 2010;34:2126–36.

18. Sutti S, Jindal A, Locatelli I, et al. Adaptive immune responses triggered by oxidative stress contribute to hepatic inflammation in NASH. Hepatology 2014;59:886–97.

19. Locatelli I, Sutti S, Vacchiano M, et al. NF-kappaB1 deficiency stimulates the progression of non-alcoholic steatohepatitis (NASH) in mice by promoting NKT-cell-mediated responses. Clin Sci (Lond) 2013;124:279–87.

20. Syn WK, Agboola KM, Swiderska M, et al. NKT-associated hedgehog and osteopontin drive fibrogenesis in non-alcoholic fatty liver disease. Gut 2012;61:1323–9.

21. Winau F, Hegasy G, Weiskirchen R, et al. Ito cells are liver-resident antigen-presenting cells for activating T cell responses. Immunity 2007;26:117–29.

22. Purohit V, Bode JC, Bode C, et al. Alcohol, intestinal bacterial growth, intestinal permeability to endotoxin, and medical consequences: summary of a symposium. Alcohol 2008;42:349–61.

23. Gustot T, Lemmers A, Moreno C, et al. Differential liver sensitization to toll-like receptor pathways in mice with alcoholic fatty liver. Hepatology 2006;43:989–1000.

24. Gao B, Seki E, Brenner DA, et al. Innate immunity in alcoholic liver disease. Am J Physiol Gastrointest Liver Physiol 2011;300:G516–25.

25. Swann JR, Want EJ, Geier FM, et al. Systemic gut microbial modulation of bile acid metabolism in host tissue compartments. Proc Natl Acad Sci U S A 2011;108(Suppl 1):4523–30.

26. Wang Z, Klipfell E, Bennett BJ, et al. Gut flora metabolism of phosphatidylcholine promotes cardiovascular disease. Nature 2011;472:57–63.

27. Cani PD, Neyrinck AM, Fava F, et al. Selective increases of bifidobacteria in gut microflora improve high-fat-diet-induced diabetes in mice through a mechanism associated with endotoxaemia. Diabetologia 2007;50:2374–83.

28. Henao-Mejia J, Elinav E, Jin C, et al. Inflammasome-mediated dysbiosis regulates progression of NAFLD and obesity. Nature 2012;482:179–85.

29. Miura K, Kodama Y, Inokuchi S, et al. Toll-like receptor 9 promotes steatohepatitis by induction of interleukin-1beta in mice. Gastroenterology 2010;139:323–34.e7.

30. Mizrahi M, Shabat Y, Ben Ya'acov A, et al. Alleviation of insulin resistance and liver damage by oral administration of Imm124-E is mediated by increased Tregs and associated with increased serum GLP-1 and adiponectin: results of a phase I/II clinical trial in NASH. J Inflamm Res 2012;5:141–50.

31. Sumida Y, Yoneda M. Current and future pharmacological therapies for NAFLD/NASH. J Gastroenterol 2018;53:362–76.

32. Rivera CA, Adegboyega P, van Rooijen N, et al. Toll-like receptor-4 signaling and Kupffer cells play pivotal roles in the pathogenesis of non-alcoholic steatohepatitis. J Hepatol 2007;47:571–9.

33. Beier JI, McClain CJ. Mechanisms and cell signaling in alcoholic liver disease. Biol Chem 2010;391:1249–64.

34. Ji C. New insights into the pathogenesis of alcohol-induced ER stress and liver diseases. Int J Hepatol 2014;2014:513787.

35. Ramirez T, Tong M, Chen WC, et al. Chronic alcohol-induced hepatic insulin resistance and endoplasmic reticulum stress ameliorated by peroxisome-proliferator activated receptor-delta agonist treatment. J Gastroenterol Hepatol 2013;28:179–87.

36. Zhang XQ, Xu CF, Yu CH, et al. Role of endoplasmic reticulum stress in the pathogenesis of nonalcoholic fatty liver disease. World J Gastroenterol 2014;20:1768–76.

37. Kammoun HL, Chabanon H, Hainault I, et al. GRP78 expression inhibits insulin and ER stress-induced SREBP-1c activation and reduces hepatic steatosis in mice. J Clin Invest 2009;119:1201–15.

38. Ota T, Gayet C, Ginsberg HN. Inhibition of apolipoprotein B100 secretion by lipid-induced hepatic endoplasmic reticulum stress in rodents. J Clin Invest 2008;118:316–32.

39. Sun LP, Seemann J, Goldstein JL, et al. Sterol-regulated transport of SREBPs from endoplasmic reticulum to Golgi: insig renders sorting signal in Scap inaccessible to COPII proteins. Proc Natl Acad Sci U S A 2007;104:6519–26.

40. Ji C, Kaplowitz N. Betaine decreases hyperhomocysteinemia, endoplasmic reticulum stress, and liver injury in alcohol-fed mice. Gastroenterology 2003;124:1488–99.

41. Ronis MJ, Korourian S, Blackburn ML, et al. The role of ethanol metabolism in development of alcoholic steatohepatitis in the rat. Alcohol 2010;44:157–69.

42. Foster DW. Malonyl-CoA: the regulator of fatty acid synthesis and oxidation. J Clin Invest 2012;122:1958–9.

43. Konerman MA, Jones JC, Harrison SA. Pharmacotherapy for NASH: current and emerging. J Hepatol 2018;68:362–75.

44. Dunn W, Shah VH. Pathogenesis of alcoholic liver disease. Clin Liver Dis 2016;20:445–56.

45. Verbeke L, Farre R, Trebicka J, et al. Obeticholic acid, a farnesoid X receptor agonist, improves portal hypertension by two distinct pathways in cirrhotic rats. Hepatology 2014;59:2286–98.

46. Mederacke I, Hsu CC, Troeger JS, et al. Fate tracing reveals hepatic stellate cells as dominant contributors to liver fibrosis independent of its aetiology. Nat Commun 2013;4:2823.

47. Dimova EY, Kietzmann T. Metabolic, hormonal and environmental regulation of plasminogen activator inhibitor-1 (PAI-1) expression: lessons from the liver. Thromb Haemost 2008;100:992–1006.

48. Alessi MC, Bastelica D, Mavri A, et al. Plasma PAI-1 levels are more strongly related to liver steatosis than to adipose tissue accumulation. Arterioscler Thromb Vasc Biol 2003;23:1262–8.

49. Luedde T, Kaplowitz N, Schwabe RF. Cell death and cell death responses in liver disease: mechanisms and clinical relevance. Gastroenterology 2014;147: 765–83.e4.

50. Di Prospero NA, Artis E, Andrade-Gordon P, et al. CCR2 antagonism in patients with type 2 diabetes mellitus: a randomized, placebo-controlled study. Diabetes Obes Metab 2014;16:1055–64.

51. Marra F, Tacke F. Roles for chemokines in liver disease. Gastroenterology 2014; 147:577–94.e1.

52. Friedman SL, Ratziu V, Harrison SA, et al. A randomized, placebo-controlled trial of cenicriviroc for treatment of nonalcoholic steatohepatitis with fibrosis. Hepatology 2018;67:1754–67.

53. Brenner C, Galluzzi L, Kepp O, et al. Decoding cell death signals in liver inflammation. J Hepatol 2013;59:583–94.

54. Loomba R, Lawitz E, Mantry PS, et al. The ASK1 inhibitor selonsertib in patients with nonalcoholic steatohepatitis: a randomized, phase 2 trial. Hepatology 2018; 67(2):549–59.

55. Moon HJ, Finney J, Ronnebaum T, et al. Human lysyl oxidase-like 2. Bioorg Chem 2014;57:231–41.

56. Henderson NC, Sethi T. The regulation of inflammation by galectin-3. Immunol Rev 2009;230:160–71.

57. Harrison SA, Marri SR, Chalasani N, et al. Randomised clinical study: GR-MD-02, a galectin-3 inhibitor, vs. placebo in patients having non-alcoholic steatohepatitis with advanced fibrosis. Aliment Pharmacol Ther 2016;44:1183–98.

58. Barreyro FJ, Holod S, Finocchietto PV, et al. The pan-caspase inhibitor Emricasan (IDN-6556) decreases liver injury and fibrosis in a murine model of non-alcoholic steatohepatitis. Liver Int 2015;35:953–66.

59. Weston CJ, Shepherd EL, Claridge LC, et al. Vascular adhesion protein-1 promotes liver inflammation and drives hepatic fibrosis. J Clin Invest 2015;125: 501–20.

Moving?

Make sure your subscription moves with you!

To notify us of your new address, find your **Clinics Account Number** (located on your mailing label above your name), and contact customer service at:

Email: journalscustomerservice-usa@elsevier.com

800-654-2452 (subscribers in the U.S. & Canada)
314-447-8871 (subscribers outside of the U.S. & Canada)

Fax number: 314-447-8029

Elsevier Health Sciences Division
Subscription Customer Service
3251 Riverport Lane
Maryland Heights, MO 63043

*To ensure uninterrupted delivery of your subscription, please notify us at least 4 weeks in advance of move.

ELSEVIER

Printed and bound by CPI Group (UK) Ltd, Croydon, CR0 4YY

03/10/2024

01040388-0015